Cardiac Doppler Ultrasound:
A Clinical Perspective

Cardiac Doppler Ultrasound:
A Clinical Perspective

Alan B. Houston, MD, FRCP(Glas.)
Consultant Paediatric Cardiologist, Royal Hospital for Sick Children, Glasgow

Iain A. Simpson, MD
Department of Medical Cardiology, Royal Infirmary, Glasgow

Wright
London   Boston   Singapore   Sydney   Toronto   Wellington

Wright
is an imprint of Butterworth Scientific

First published 1988

© **Butterworth & Co. (Publishers) Ltd, 1988**

British Library Cataloguing in Publication Data

Houston, Alan B.
    Cardiac doppler ultrasound.
    1. Man. Heart. Diagnosis. Doppler
    echocardiography
    I. Title   II. Simpson, Iain A.
    616.1'207543

ISBN 0-723-60995-0

Library of Congress Cataloging in Publication Data

Cardiac doppler ultrasound : a clinical perspective/[edited by] Alan
    B. Houston, Iain A. Simpson.
        p. cm.
    ISBN 0-723-60995-0
    1. Doppler echocardiography.   2. Heart–Diseases–Diagnosis.
    3. Heart–Valves–Diseases–Diagnosis.   I. Houston, Alan B.
    II. Simpson, Iain A.
    [DNLM: 1. Echocardiography.   2. Heart Defects, Congenital
    RC683.5.U5C364   1988
    616.1'207543–dc 19
    DNLM/DLC   88-5548

Photoset by Butterworths Litho Preparation Department
Printed in Great Britain at the University Press, Cambridge

Preface

The development of Doppler ultrasound has given a new and exciting perspective to non-invasive cardiovascular diagnosis. Over the past five years spectral Doppler ultrasound has been extensively applied to the majority of cardiac lesions in both adult and paediatric cardiology. Comprehensive textbooks on Doppler ultrasound are available but they do not necessarily provide a guide to the practical application of the technique and, to our knowledge, none has placed Doppler ultrasound in clinical perspective to conventional non-invasive assessment. This book has attempted to define the present role of cardiac Doppler ultrasound in clinical practice, highlighting not only areas where it has established a significant clinical value but also the problems which may be encountered in its application.

Persons actively involved in echocardiography may currently be introducing and developing Doppler ultrasound in their institutions and this textbook has been designed to provide them with a guide to the practical application of cardiac Doppler, a perspective to its clinical value, and an insight into its problems and pitfalls. As the technique has become widely available other cardiologists and general physicians will have become aware of Doppler ultrasound and we hope that they will find this textbook useful in outlining the areas of cardiology where Doppler ultrasound can prove a valuable adjunct to conventional investigative techniques and what reliance can be placed on the Doppler investigation, even if they have no particular expertise in this.

We have assembled a group of authors, each of whom not only has substantial expertise and personal involvement in performing Doppler examinations, but also applies the results of Doppler ultrasound examination in daily clinical practice and is therefore qualified to comment on its clinical value. This means that each author's comments will be personal ones based on individual experience: as a result agreement with some of the statements in this book may not be universal, but these opinions are made by persons in the forefront of Doppler research, with considerable experience in the use of cardiac Doppler, and well qualified to make them.

The book does not attempt to provide a comprehensive approach to all the possible applications of Doppler ultrasound or to provide a comprehensive source of Doppler references. Other books exist which more adequately fulfill this role, and in particular the text of Hatle and Angelsen, *Doppler Ultrasound in Cardiology* must be considered to be the major reference on the subject. Since colour Doppler flow mapping has only been introduced recently the clinical role of this technique is far from established and the majority of the text will, by necessity, deal with spectral Doppler and its more established role in clinical cardiological practice. The authors already find colour Doppler of considerable clinical value and the impact of this dynamic technique will expand considerably over the next few years as its role becomes more established. Therefore we have included a chapter on the principles of colour Doppler flow mapping and discuss its potential clinical role in addition to the inclusion of colour Doppler within the main chapters where the authors deem it to be of particular clinical importance, even at present.

Persons developing their skills in performing and interpreting Doppler examinations will often encounter more questions than answers. We hope that the practical aspect of this textbook and the emphasis on associated problems and pitfalls will provide answers to at least some of the questions. However, not all problems can be listed in this book without diluting the important perspective of the clinical value of cardiac Doppler ultrasound. We would therefore actively encourage anyone who encounters a problem or has a question which is not covered in this textbook to contact the Editors who will do their best to clarify the problem.

Alan B. Houston
Iain A. Simpson

Contributors

Walter J. Duncan, MD, FRCP(C)
University of Saskatchewan, Saskatoon, Saskatchewan, Canada S7N 0X0

Donald J. Hagler, MD
Mayo Medical School, Mayo Clinic, Rochester MN 55905, USA

Alan B. Houston, MD, FRCP(Glas)
Royal Hospital for Sick Children, Glasgow G13 1QD, UK

Graham J. Leech, MA
St George's Hospital Medical School, London SW17, UK

A. P. G. Mayala, MD
Faculty of Medicine, University of Dar-es-Salaam, Tanzania; and Thoraxcenter, Eramus University and Academic Hospital, Rotterdam, The Netherlands

J. Roelandt, MD, FACC
Thoraxcenter, Eramus University and Academic Hospital, Rotterdam, The Netherlands

Iain A. Simpson, MD
University of California Medical Center, San Diego, California 92103, USA; and Glasgow Royal Infirmary, Glasgow, UK

Terje Skjaerpe, MD
Regional Hospital, 7000 Trondheim, Norway

George R. Sutherland, MB ChB, MRCP(UK)
Southampton General Hospital, Southampton, UK

Neil Wilson, MB, BS, DCH, MRCP(UK)
Killingbeck Hospital, Leeds, UK

Contents

1

Analysis of blood velocity with Doppler ultrasound

Graham Leech

Basic concepts of ultrasound imaging

If a disturbance is initiated in a medium in which the constituent particles have freedom of movement, some of the energy in the disturbance is transmitted through the medium in the form of compression waves. The disturbance initially displaces those particles adjacent to it, but they soon collide with their neighbours, passing on most of their energy and bouncing back towards their original positions. Through rapid repetition of this process a wave of disturbance is propagated through the medium. The bunching up of particles as they collide, and subsequent separation as they rebound causes local fluctuations in the pressure within the medium. The higher the amplitude of the pressure changes, the greater the energy carried by the wave. The velocity at which the wave travels is characteristic of the medium and for soft body tissues such as muscle, fat and blood, the value is about 1540 m/s.

If a succession of waves is generated by a vibrating source, a series of regular waves, comprising alternating pressure peaks and troughs, is generated. The distance between successive pressure peaks is the wavelength; the number of peaks passing a given point per second is the frequency. Propagation velocity, frequency and wavelength are linked by the relationship:

propagation velocity = wavelength × frequency

Thus at a frequency of 1000 Hz (Hz = Hertz, the unit of frequency equal to one wave/s), the wavelength in soft body tissues is 154 cm. Common sense dictates that such a large wavelength is unsuitable for obtaining information about a heart valve, which is less than 1 mm thick. Since propagation velocity has a fixed value for a given medium, it follows that it is necessary to increase the frequency to several megahertz (1 MHz = 1 000 000 cycles/s) in order to achieve wavelengths of under 1 mm.

The frequency chosen for clinical purposes is a compromise between the need to use a wavelength small enough to provide fine detail in images and the fact that an increase in the frequency impairs transmission of energy due to absorption and scattering by small imperfections in the transmission medium and limits the maximum depth from which echoes can be detected. With current technology a frequency of 3.5 MHz is typically used to image adult hearts, at which the wavelength is 0.44 mm. In children, depth of penetration is not so important and improved image quality is achieved by increasing the frequency to 5 or 7 MHz, giving wavelengths of 0.31 and 0.22 mm respectively. Such frequencies are called *ultrasound* since they greatly exceed the upper limit of the frequency range which the human ear can detect (about 15 kHz).

Ultrasound can easily be generated and detected by employing the piezo-electric properties of crystals. A slice of a suitable crystal (usually lead zirconate titanate, a synthetic ceramic) is sandwiched between two thin metal foil electrodes. When a voltage is applied to the electrodes the electric field stresses the crystal lattice, causing it to change its shape. This disturbs the medium surrounding the crystal and initiates a short burst of compression waves. The piezo-electric effect is reversible: when the crystal is struck by a wave it is slightly deformed and this generates a small electrical impulse which can be detected and amplified to indicate the arrival of the wave. A piezo-electric crystal can thus be used as a *transducer*, converting electrical energy into mechanical energy and vice versa.

Since both light and sound are examples of wave motion, they share many physical properties. For example, when ultrasound waves encounter an extensive boundary between two different transmission media, some of the incident energy is reflected and the path of the remainder is deflected by refraction as it crosses the interface. The reflections are said to be *specular* (mirror-like) and the angle between the path of the incident waves and the normal to the plane of the interface is equal to the corresponding angle of the reflected portion. The fact that light can be formed into a narrow beam, whereas audible sound waves spread out to fill a room is due to the enormous difference in their wavelengths, approximately 0.0005 mm for light compared with several metres for sound. Ultrasound, having a wavelength of about 0.5 mm lies between these two extremes. Unlike sound, it can be directed in a fairly well-defined beam towards a target, but it cannot be focused as sharply as light. As can be seen from *Figure 1.1* an ultrasound beam comprises a central main beam, surrounded by a series of secondary beams called *side-lobes*.

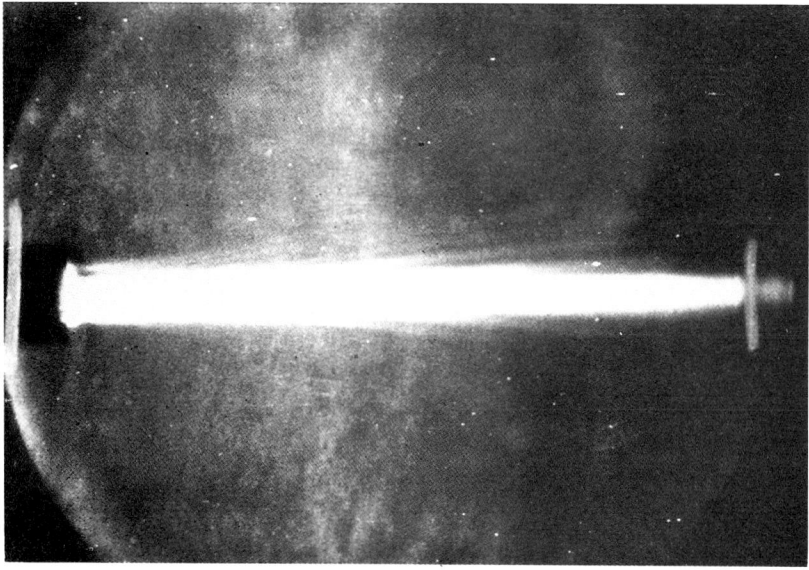

Figure 1.1 A photograph taken by the Schlieren technique showing an ultrasound beam passing through water from a transducer at the left to a target at the right. The width of the main beam is approximately that of the transducer and it is surrounded by secondary side-lobes

These illuminate structures other than the primary target and are a troublesome source of artefacts on ultrasound images. Some improvement can be obtained by narrowing the main beam using a plastic focusing lens.

The basis of echocardiographic imaging is to direct a series of very short pulses of ultrasound into the heart from a transducer positioned on the chest wall in such a way that the ultrasound beam avoids ribs, sternum and lungs, all of which are effectively impenetrable to ultrasound in the adult. As each pulse travels through the heart it encounters a series of tissue interfaces, mainly between blood and muscle or connective tissues. At each interface a small proportion of the incident energy is reflected. If the beam crosses the interface at right angles, the reflections return along the same path to the transducer, where their arrival can be detected. Since the propagation velocity is known, the distance of each reflector can be determined from the time delay between pulse transmission and the arrival of its echo; the further away the reflector, the longer the time for the echo to return.

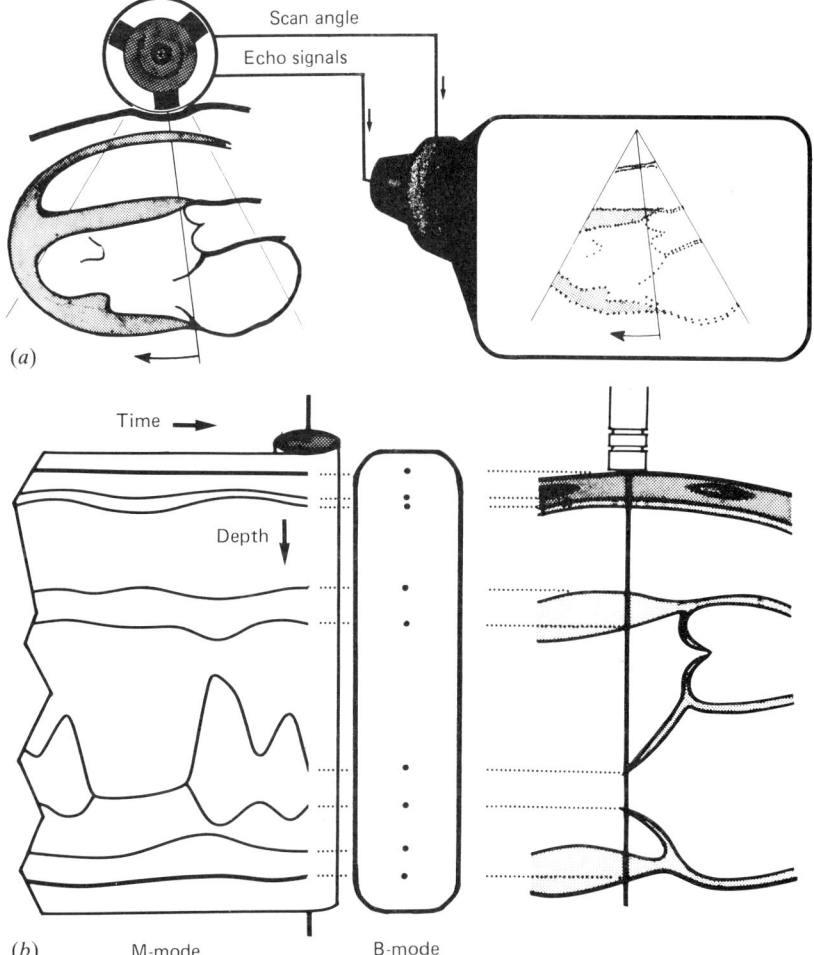

Figure 1.2 Diagrams showing (a) how a two-dimensional image is formed using a mechanical scanning system and (b) how an M-mode recording is made

Once all the echoes of interest have returned, another pulse can be transmitted. After electronic processing, the echo signals can be displayed in two ways. If the direction of the ultrasound beam is swept rapidly across the heart, and returning echoes are shown as variations in brightness of a beam swept in a corresponding manner across the face of a cathode-ray, an image of the section of the heart scanned by the beam can be built up (*Figure 1.2a*). This is essentially similar to the way in which radar information from rotating scanners at airports and on ships is displayed. Alternatively, the ultrasound beam can be aimed in a fixed direction and the displacements of the echoes from cardiac structures as they move can be recorded on light-sensitive film, known as an *M-mode* echocardiogram (*Figure 1.2b*).

Detection of blood flow by ultrasound: continuous wave Doppler

As stated above, ultrasound images are derived from echoes generated at extensive interfaces between different types of tissue. However, body tissues are not homogeneous and contain many structures too small to generate specular echoes. The ultrasound beam sets these vibrating and they act as miniature sources, radiating waves in all directions, like the ripples after a stone is dropped into a pond. Most of this energy is lost, but a small proportion returns to the transducer as *back-scattered* echoes and is one of the sources of *noise* on echocardiographic images. For imaging purposes, it is common practice to remove most of these signals electronically. Red blood cells generate back-scattered echoes: an individual red blood cell could never generate a detectable echo, but the summated scattered energy from the millions of cells in a blood vessel is sufficient to be recorded.

If the blood is moving relative to the direction of the ultrasound beam the frequency of the returning echoes differs slightly from that of the transmitted waves as a consequence of the Doppler effect. This well-known phenomenon is generally associated with movement of a wave source. When the source moves towards an observer its emitted waves are compressed, shortening the wavelength and increasing the frequency, and when the source is receding the wavelength is increased and frequency lowered. It was first postulated in 1842 by Christian Doppler, an Austrian mathematician who observed that the line spectra of distant stars are shifted slightly towards the red (longer wavelength) end of the spectrum and deduced that the stars must be moving away from the solar system at enormous speeds. It does not matter whether the observer is moving towards the source or vice versa as it is the relative velocity which produces the frequency shift. The Doppler effect also modifies the frequency of waves reflected from a moving target, which can be considered to be a receiver, which then re-transmits the waves. If the target moves towards the source, the frequency it receives is increased. Echoes arriving back at the source are further increased in frequency by the fact that the *transmitter* is moving towards it. The total frequency shift produced by a reflector is thus double that if it were either a transmitter or receiver alone. If the motion of the reflector is not along the axis of wave propagation, only that component of its velocity in the direction of the ultrasound beam axis can modify the wave frequency.

The principle of using the Doppler effect to measure blood flow velocity with ultrasound is shown in *Figure 1.3*. Two piezo-electric crystals are used, one to

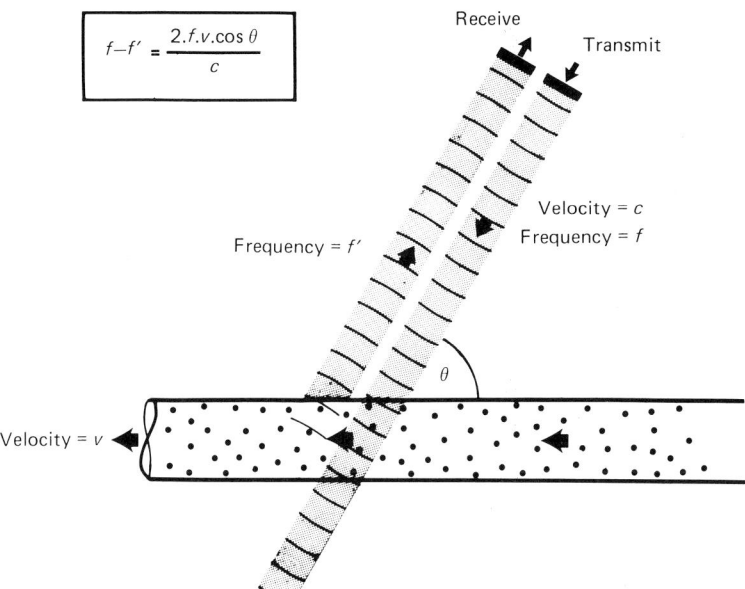

$$f - f' = \frac{2.f.v.\cos\theta}{c}$$

Receive

Transmit

Velocity = c
Frequency = f

Frequency = f'

θ

Velocity = v

Figure 1.3 The Doppler principle. f and f' = transmitted and received frequencies respectively; c = ultrasound propagation velocity; V = blood flow velocity; θ = angle between ultrasound beam and direction of flow

transmit a continuous series of ultrasonic waves across the moving blood stream and the other to receive back-scattered echoes. The difference between transmitted frequency, f, and received frequency, f' is given by:

$$f - f' = \frac{2.f.v.\cos\theta}{c}.$$

where v is the blood velocity, c the propagation velocity and θ the angle between the beam axis and flow direction. The frequency shift $(f - f')$ is called the *Doppler frequency* and, if the other terms in the equation are kept constant, is directly proportional to the blood velocity, so in Doppler jargon the terms *frequency* and *velocity* can be treated as synonymous. This technique is called continuous wave (CW) Doppler.

It can be seen from *Figure 1.3* that there is a fundamental dichotomy between the requirements for imaging a blood vessel and measuring the blood velocity. For the former the ultrasound beam should strike it at right angles ($\theta = 90°$) but the blood flow has no velocity component in this direction. To obtain the maximum flow signal θ should be 0°, but this makes it difficult to image the vessel as its walls do not generate clear echoes. For any intermediate angle the value of θ must be known. Thus although imaging and Doppler studies are performed as part of a single examination, it is necessary to treat cardiac imaging and analysis of blood flow as separate procedures; for the former the beam is directed to obtain specular echoes from the major tissue interfaces, whereas for the latter the objective is to try to align the beam as closely as possible with the direction of the blood flow being studied, even if this means that the quality of the associated cardiac image is adversely affected. Provided this angle can be kept below 15°, for which cos θ = 0.97, the velocity error is negligible.

Characteristics of blood flow

Precise mathematical modelling of blood flow in the heart and great arteries is almost impossible. Although some insight into the nature of blood flow can be obtained by applying methods developed by engineers and physicists for analysis of fluid flow in pipes, the application of these to the cardiovascular system introduces a number of errors due to the fact that blood has special properties, and arteries are not rigid and do not have smooth walls. The following discussion can therefore be taken only as a very rough approximation to the truth. In *Figure 1.3* all the red cells are shown to be moving at the same velocity, but this is not true because there is friction between the blood and the vessel walls and the blood itself has viscosity. As a result, velocity is greatest in the centre of the vessel, and at the edges friction slows it down so that the layer actually in contact with the wall does not move at all. *Figure 1.4* shows cross-sections through two pipes, with the velocity at each point indicated by the length of the arrows. The curve joining the arrow tips is called the *velocity profile*. In the narrow pipe, the proportion of flow affected by wall friction (the *boundary layer*) is relatively greater and results in a sharply pointed velocity profile, whereas in the wide pipe the profile is much blunter. The highest velocity, in the centre of the pipe, is called the *peak velocity*. If all the fluid had the same velocity, the volume flowing through the pipe per second could be calculated by multiplying this velocity by the cross-sectional area of the pipe. In practice for this calculation it is necessary to use the average of all the velocities present across the area of the pipe, which is called the *space-averaged mean*. The total range of velocities present, from zero at the edges to the peak in the centre, is called the *velocity spectrum*. Another term used to characterize velocity profiles is the *modal velocity*, which is the value possessed by the greatest number of fluid particles. In the wide pipe, with flat velocity profile, the majority of the velocity spectrum is concentrated in a narrow range, with very little contribution from the edges, so the peak, space-averaged mean and modal values are nearly the same and the majority of the velocity spectrum is concentrated close to the peak. In the narrow pipe there is a more even distribution of velocities across the spectrum, and the mean value is significantly lower than the peak.

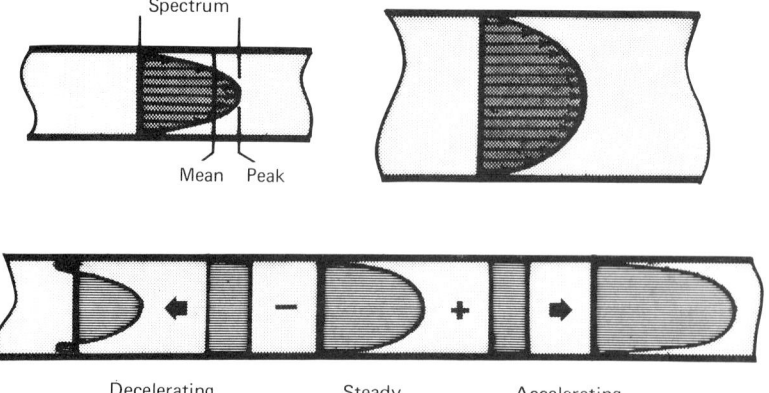

Figure 1.4 Diagrams showing flow velocity profiles in a narrow pipe (top left), and a wide pipe (top right). Modification of the flow profile by acceleration or deceleration is shown below

For arteries, the above considerations are further complicated by the fact that the blood flow is pulsatile. Not only do the peak and mean velocities vary, but the combined effects of viscous friction and inertia of the blood mass as it is accelerated and decelerated cause the velocity profile to change throughout the cardiac cycle. The contribution of acceleration or deceleration is to add a changing velocity, increasing or decreasing the steady flow profile, but which acts uniformly across the tube area, as it is unaffected by friction. The sum of the two velocity profiles results in a flatter profile during acceleration and a greater velocity spread during deceleration, with flow near the edges actually reversing (*see Figure 1.4*). When flow is pulsatile, the average rate is determined by first taking the mean over the area of the pipe at a particular time (space-averaged mean), and further averaging this over the period of an integral number of pumping cycles. This is termed the *time-averaged mean velocity* and, when multiplied by the pipe cross-sectional area, gives the average volumetric flow rate, e.g. left ventricular stroke output when applied to flow in the ascending aorta.

Displaying and recording velocity data: spectral analysis

To provide the maximum potential clinical value it is necessary to display information derived from Doppler frequency shifts caused by moving blood in such a way that all the flow characteristics can be analysed. As shown above the blood cells in a vessel or cardiac chamber do not all travel at the same velocity. Moreover, the ultrasound beam in a continuous wave Doppler mode may pass across more than one chamber or vessel before attenuation weakens it too much to return detectable signals. Each velocity component generates its own Doppler frequency, so the signal detected by the receiving crystal comprises a very complex spectrum of frequencies and amplitudes. It is like sitting in an auditorium listening to an orchestra with 90 instruments playing many different notes, each at various intensities.

In Doppler terms, each velocity component is represented by a particular frequency and the intensity at each frequency, which is related to the sum of the scattered echoes from the individual red cells, indicates the volume of blood having that particular velocity.

A trained musician can listen to a chord of several notes and identify each one correctly. When the complex wave comprising the chord arrives at the eardrum and is transmitted to the cochlea, it excites different groups of sensory hairs, each responding to a particular frequency, and which convey to the brain the characteristics of the sound and enable it to separate the notes present. This is essentially the task performed electronically and at high speed by the spectral analyser in Doppler apparatus. Most commercial machines employ a fast Fourier transform (FFT) analyser, named after a French mathematician who showed that it is possible to break down almost any complex wave into a series of constituents comprising a fundamental frequency and a series of harmonics, whose frequencies are integral multiples of that of the fundamental. The FFT analyser effectively comprises a bank of filters (usually 64), each tuned to a different narrow frequency band. Over a brief period (typically 10 ms) the incoming waves are passed through the filters and the amount of energy each detects is stored in memory cells, like a postman sorting a heap of letters. At the end of the analysis period the contents of each cell are shown on the display as a vertical row of pixels, the density of each of

8

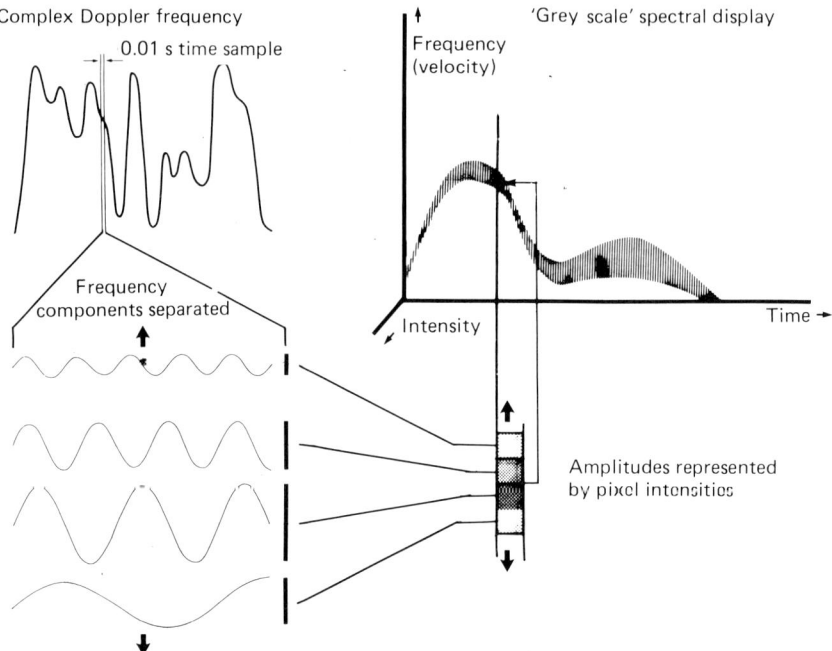

Complex Doppler frequency

0.01 s time sample

Frequency
components separated

'Grey scale' spectral display

Frequency
(velocity)

Intensity

Time →

Amplitudes represented
by pixel intensities

Figure 1.5 Diagram showing how a fast Fourier transform (FFT) spectral analyser separates the components of a complex Doppler frequency and displays their amplitudes as pixel intensities

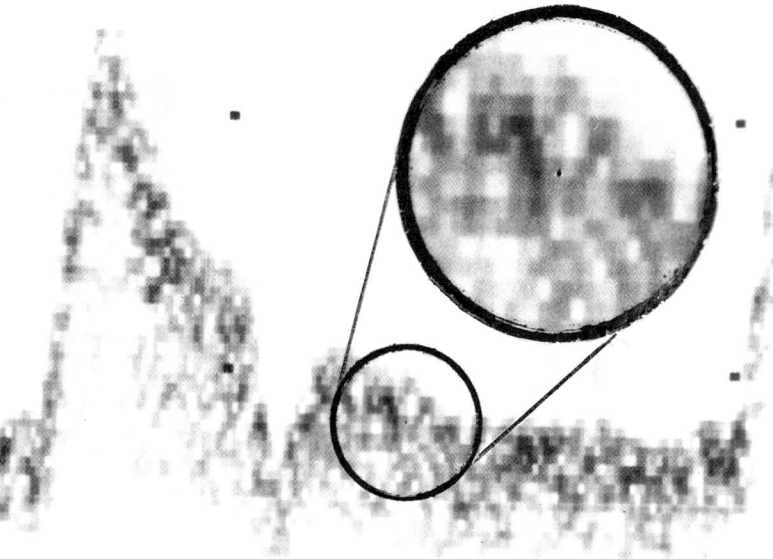

Figure 1.6 Spectral recording of normal aortic arch flow, with magnified section showing the pixel structure

which indicates the accumulated energy in the corresponding frequency band (*Figures 1.5* and *1.6*). A horizontal line marks zero velocity. The blackness of the pixel immediately above it shows the amount of blood having the lowest Doppler frequency (= velocity) during the analysis period; the pixel above that shows the amount in the next velocity band, and so on. The pixel stores are then erased ready for the next computation. A 10 ms analysis period corresponds to 100 measurements/s.

From this a number of parameters can be obtained for use in the calculation of blood flow and pressure gradient parameters:

the *peak velocity* at any instant is indicated by uppermost limit of the dark region
the *modal velocity* is shown by the pixel having the darkest grey level
the *mean velocity* can be approximated as the centre of the dark band (or can be calculated electronically).

Pulsed wave Doppler

Continuous wave Doppler permits quantification of blood velocity, from which indices of cardiac performance and pressure gradients across stenotic valves can be derived. However, because the waves are transmitted in a continuous stream it is not possible to identify the time interval between transmission of a particular wave and arrival of its echo, so continuous wave Doppler cannot provide any structural information. Furthermore, any moving structure in the path of the beam returns a Doppler frequency, up to the point where depth is so great that the beam becomes too attenuated to allow these to be detected. In cases where there is more than one high velocity jet, e.g. in the left ventricle in the presence of both mitral stenosis and aortic regurgitation, both Doppler spectra are superimposed, with the possibility of one masking the other. It would clearly be very useful to obtain Doppler information from a specific location within the cardiovascular system, with the location identified on a conventional echocardiographic image. This is possible using the technique of pulsed wave (PW) Doppler, first introduced by Perroneau in 1969, and shortly afterwards by Baker. Since then, developments in pulsed wave and continuous wave Doppler have proceeded concurrently, but unfortunately the devotees of each method have tended to foster rivalry between them, rather than promoting their complementary features.

Referring to *Figure 1.7*, two-dimensional and M-mode images are derived from high intensity specular echoes but between these are much lower intensity back-scattered echoes arising from blood cells. A small *time-gate* is positioned at a selected point along the beam path. Its distance from the transducer is determined by choosing the time delay following pulse transmission at which the gate is opened (i.e. the time taken for the sound beam to reach the chosen point and return to the transducer). The frequencies in the echoes returning while the gate is open are compared with that of the transmitted pulse and their Doppler shifts analysed to indicate the blood velocity spectrum at the chosen depth. The time aperture is called the *sample volume*; it can be moved to any chosen site on the two-dimensional image and its depth and position are indicated on the display by electronic markers superimposed on the cursor used for deriving M-modes from the two-dimensional images. It is important to remember that the sample volume is a transverse slice of the ultrasound beam; it is three-dimensional and comprises not only a section of the main ultrasound beam, but also its associated side-lobes.

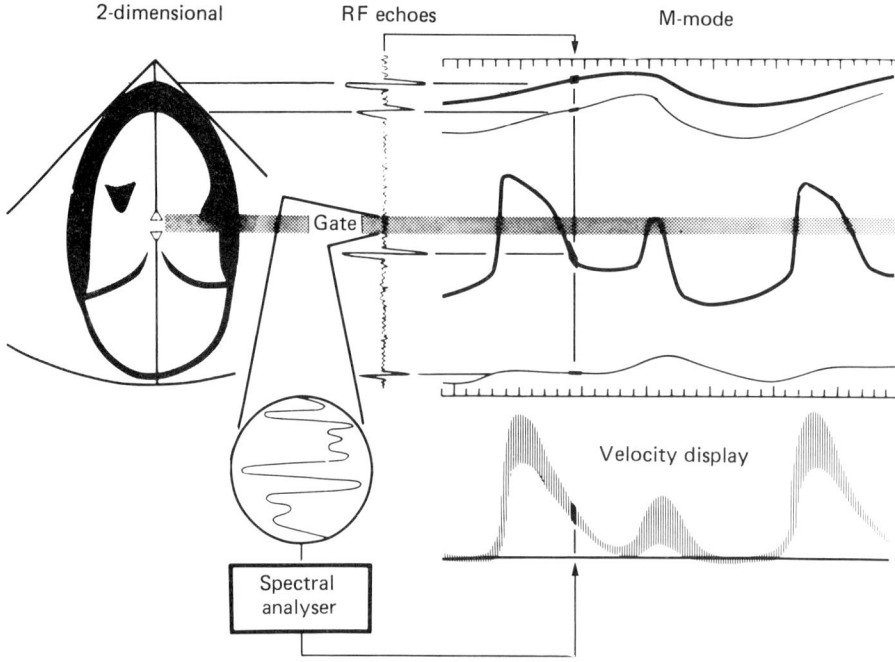

Figure 1.7 Derivation of M-mode and blood velocity recordings from a two-dimensional image using pulsed Doppler

While its length is precisely controlled by the setting of the time-gate, its width increases with distance from the transducer as the beam spreads out. The electronic markers used to indicate the position of the sample volume on the display thus provide only an indication of its position and length and not its width (*Figure 1.8*). It is important to remember this when considering, for example, the accuracy of Doppler *mapping* of regurgitant jets in the left atrium, which is typically 10–15 cm from the transducer and where the overall width of the main beam plus side-lobes can easily be 3 cm.

In order to generate an image, each time a burst of ultrasound is transmitted the transmitter has to wait while it travels to and returns from the target before sending out another burst of ultrasound. The deeper the target the longer between each burst and vice versa. The rate at which the bursts of ultrasound are sent out is the *pulse repetition frequency* (PRF). This should not be confused with the *ultrasound frequency* (termed *f* in the Doppler equation of *Figure 1.3*) which is a property determined by the characteristics of the transducer crystal.

Aliasing

Pulsed wave Doppler overcomes the problem of defining the location at which flow is analysed, but unfortunately it suffers from a different, serious limitation, to understand which it is necessary to introduce some basic concepts of information theory. Since the ultrasound beam now consists of a series of brief pulses, each a few microseconds long and separated by intervals of about 300 μs, blood velocity

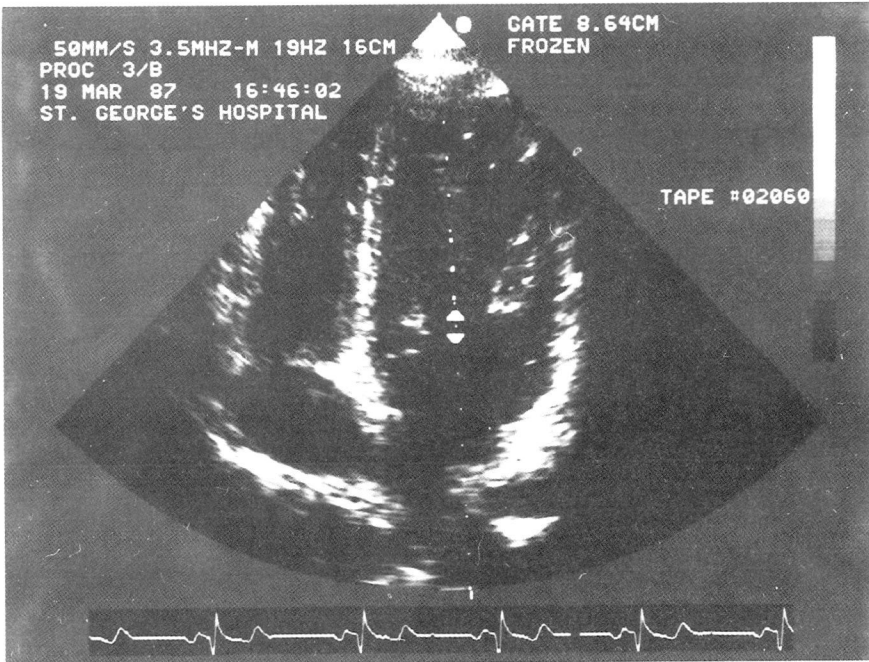

(a)

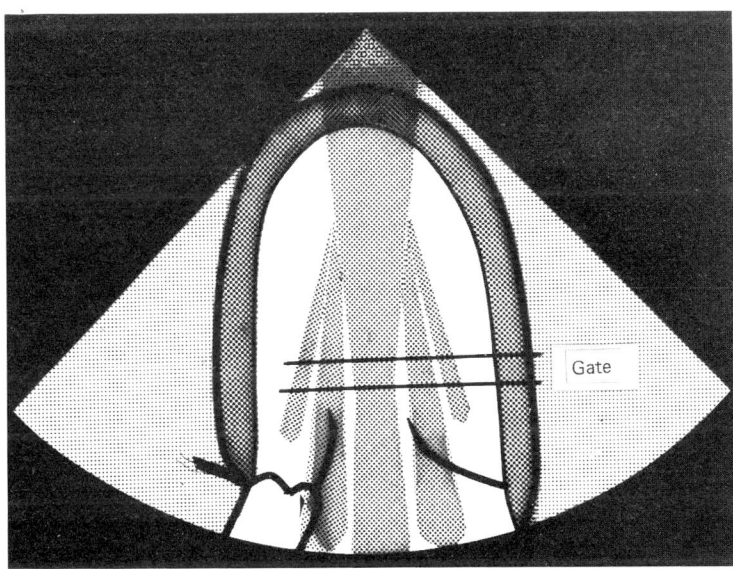

(b)

Figure 1.8 The depiction of the sample volume on the two-dimensional image (a) and a diagram of the actual beam dimensions and the sample volume (b)

data are acquired in the form of a series of very brief 'snapshots'. A similar situation exists in a movie camera, where each opening of the shutter lasts for less than 1/100 s and the exposures are spaced at about 1/25 s intervals. In the familiar 'Western' movie, as the stagecoach moves off the spoked wheels rotate normally at first but as its speed increases they suddenly appear to be rotating very fast backwards. With further increase in speed the backward motion slows down, stops, and rotation again appears to be in the normal direction. To understand how this effect is produced, consider a wheel with a single radial spoke. If the wheel rotates slowly the angular displacement of the spoke between successive film shutter openings is small and no confusion concerning its motion arises. As it speeds up the angle it turns through between successive exposures increases until eventually it becomes exactly one half-circle (180°). At this point one exposure occurs when the spoke is in the 12 o'clock position, the next at 6 o'clock, the next at 12 o'clock, and so on. To the observer, the position of the spoke alternates between the two extremes and it is impossible to identify the direction of rotation. With further increase in speed the rotation between exposures becomes greater than 180°, giving the impression that the wheel is rotating in the opposite direction. As the rotation per exposure approaches a full circle, the wheel appears to slow down until, at exactly 360° per exposure, it appears to be stationary. Further increase in rotational speed repeats this entire process. This is an example of a phenomenon called *aliasing* and can be represented graphically (*Figure 1.9*).

It will be seen from the above analysis that the wheel's motion is recorded correctly by the intermittent exposures of the movie camera only when it rotates less than 180° per exposure or, put another way, when at least two exposures are made per rotation. This is a fundamental principle of sampling theory, first stated by Nyquist, namely that the maximum frequency that can be detected by intermittent sampling is equal to half the sampling rate. When applied to pulsed wave Doppler it means that the maximum Doppler frequency which can be detected without aliasing is equal to half the PRF. If the blood velocity exceeds the value for which the Doppler frequency is 1/2 (PRF), called the *Nyquist limit*, the

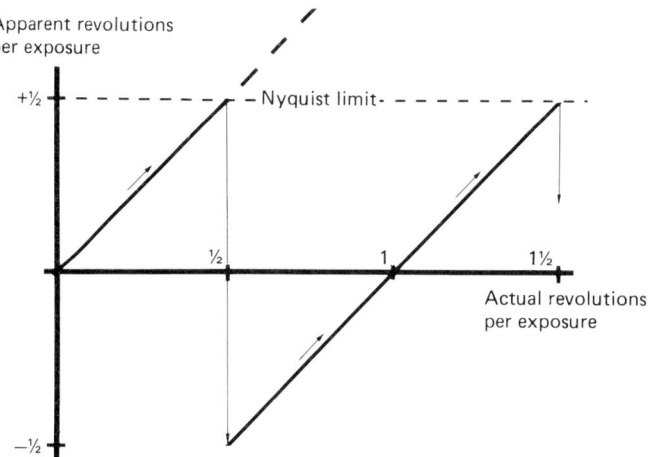

Figure 1.9 Graphic representation of aliasing associated with filming a rotating wheel (*see* text). Correct representation of the direction and speed of rotation is only possible below the Nyquist limit, i.e. when the revolution frequency is less than half the exposure frequency

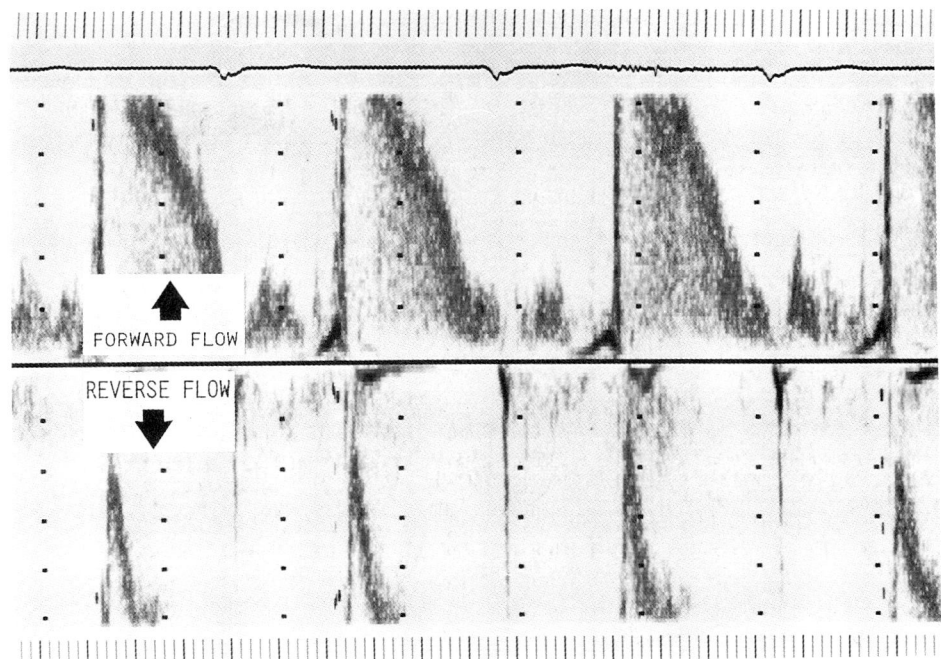

Figure 1.10 Pulsed wave recording of mitral valve flow velocity showing mild aliasing

highest velocity components of the spectral display are cut off and shown on the negative velocity portion of the display (*Figure 1.10*). When the Doppler frequency is equal to the PRF the velocity is shown as having zero value (corresponding to 360° wheel rotation per exposure). Up to this point, the true peak velocity can still be estimated by adding together the positive and negative sections of the display (which can be achieved electronically by moving the baseline to the bottom of the scale), but if velocity exceeds this there is complete wrap-around and in extreme cases it can be difficult to tell in which direction the blood is flowing. Even mild aliasing distorts computations of mean or modal velocity values.

Aliasing presents a very real practical limitation to the use of pulsed wave Doppler for quantification of blood velocities. Taking for example a work depth of 10 cm, for which the round trip echo delay is 155 μs, the maximum possible pulse rate is 6540/s. The maximum detectable Doppler frequency without aliasing is therefore 3225 Hz. Putting this value into the Doppler equation of *Figure 1.3*, for zero angular offset at an ultrasound frequency of 3.5 MHz the maximum detectable blood velocity is 0.71 m/s, a value which is below that of normal aortic ejection velocity. There are three possible ways in which this limit can be increased.

First, if the angle θ is deliberately made fairly large the maximum measurable velocity can be increased by a factor of $1/\cos\theta$ but, unless the angle is known precisely (and remembering that we are dealing with a three-dimensional system), this introduces significant errors, as shown below. Second, the ultrasound frequency can be reduced. At 2.25 MHz the velocity limit increases to 1.1 m/s and at 1.5 MHz it is 1.7 m/s. Lowering the frequency degrades image quality but the Doppler information is better. Finally, if depth can be reduced the velocity limit increases since the pulse rate can be increased proportionally. This is often not possible in practice due to limitations of imaging windows and the need to align the ultrasound beam with blood flow, but it points out the principle that, because maximum measurable velocity is inversely proportional to pulse rate, and hence range, for each value of ultrasound frequency the onset of aliasing occurs at a fixed value of: range × blood velocity.

In practice, pulsed wave Doppler is useful for any application involving detection of abnormal flow and where the actual value of the blood velocity is not important, for example diagnosis of mild aortic regurgitation, but if velocities above 1–2 m/s are present, continuous wave Doppler is generally necessary to provide quantitative data.

Further reading

HATLE, L. and ANGELSEN, B. (1985) *Doppler Ultrasound in Cardiology: Physical Principles and Clinical Applications,* 2nd edn. Philadelphia: Lea and Febiger

McDONALD, D. A. (1974) *Blood Flow in Arteries,* 2nd edn. London: Edward Arnold

2

Technical considerations in the application of Doppler ultrasound

Graham Leech

The derivation of haemodynamic parameters from Doppler data

Stroke distance and volume flow

On a recording of spectral flow data such as shown in *Figure 1.6*, the dimensions in the plane of the paper represent time on the abscissa and velocity on the ordinate. An area in the plane of the paper therefore has the dimensions of time × velocity, or distance. This concept can be applied to measure flow rates at selected points in the cardiovascular system, e.g. the ascending aorta (*Figure 2.1*). A Doppler recording of blood velocity is made from the suprasternal notch. The area under the systolic ejection portion of the curve, which can be measured by planimetry, is called the *stroke distance*, and in physical terms represents the distance up the aorta which a particular layer of blood moves during one cardiac cycle. If the cross-sectional area of the aorta is measured separately from an echocardiographic recording obtained from the parasternal region, the product of aortic area × stroke distance is the volume of the cylinder of blood ejected during one cycle, or the *stroke volume*.

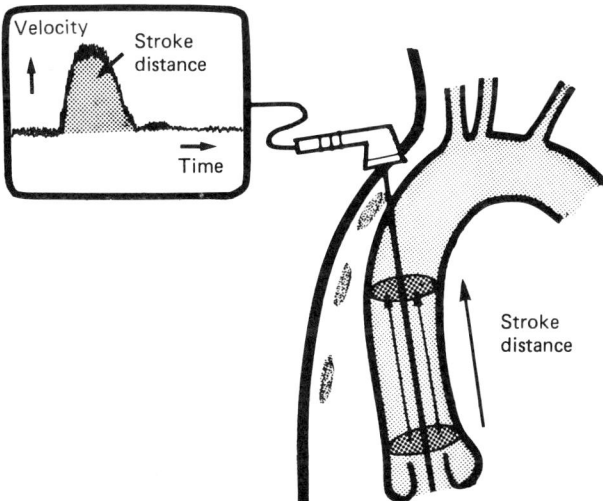

Figure 2.1 The computation of stroke distance from a spectral velocity recording and its physiological significance when applied to flow in the ascending aorta

It is important to emphasize that the value of velocity used for this purpose should not be the top of the spectral band, which corresponds to the instantaneous peak velocity, but the space-averaged mean velocity, which for laminar flow in a large artery is almost the same as the modal velocity. If peak velocity is used, the area under the curve will be overestimated by a significant factor. Some commercial machines provide a facility for displaying modal and/or mean velocity, either separately or superimposed on the spectral display.

Turbulence: Reynolds' number

In 1883, Osborne Reynolds studied the flow of water in pipes by injecting fine streams of dye into the water. He observed that at relatively low velocities the flow was stable, or streamlined, but at high velocities the flow became chaotic, or turbulent. He found that turbulent flow occurred if Reynolds' number (equal to the product of the liquid density, velocity and pipe diameter, divided by the liquid viscosity) exceeded a certain value. Under ideal experimental conditions, the critical value of Reynolds' number below which turbulence is never found is about 2000, and it is possible to maintain laminar flow up to values of 10 000 or more. At values of Reynolds' number above 20 000, flow becomes completely chaotic, with random velocities in all directions superimposed on the overall mean flow. Although for the reasons stated earlier, fluid theory is only approximately applicable to pulsatile blood flow, it is interesting to note that inserting approximate values for blood viscosity (10^{-2} Paschal·s) and density (1.06×10^{3} kg/m^{3}) yields a Reynolds' number of 530 for an artery 0.5 cm in diameter and blood velocity 1 m/s, whereas at the same velocity in the aorta, diameter 2.5 cm, it is 2650. This is in accord with clinical experience that a small increase in flow velocity in major arteries due to pyrexia, anaemia or pregnancy frequently generates enough turbulence to produce an audible murmur.

On a spectral recording, laminar flow is indicated by a relatively narrow dark band, showing that the majority of the fluid is travelling at similar velocities. In contrast, turbulent flow is represented by a much broader band, with much higher peak velocity, very low or even negative velocities present, and a more even grey shade indicating that flow is divided evenly across the complete velocity range (*Figure 2.2*).

Since fluids are incompressible, if there is flow in a rigid pipe the diameter of which varies, the instantaneous flow rates must be identical at all points along the pipe. Therefore, in the case of steady laminar flow, at points where the cross-sectional areas are A1, A2 and A3 and the mean velocities V1, V2 and V3, it follows that A1 × V1 = A2 × V2 = A3 × V3. This is a useful concept to apply to the blood circulation since, for example, in absence of any shunt lesion the mean flow rates across the aortic and pulmonary valves are the same, so if both velocities can be measured and the area of one valve is known, the effective orifice area of the other can be calculated. Since area is in turn proportional to the square of tube diameter, the relationship can be written as:

$$(d1)^2 \times V1 = (d2)^2 \times V2$$

Thus, if the diameter of the pipe halves, its area is reduced by a factor of four and the velocity must increase by a factor of four. Since Reynolds' number is proportional to the product of diameter and velocity, the net effect of reducing the diameter is to increase Reynolds' number by a factor of two. A reduction in blood

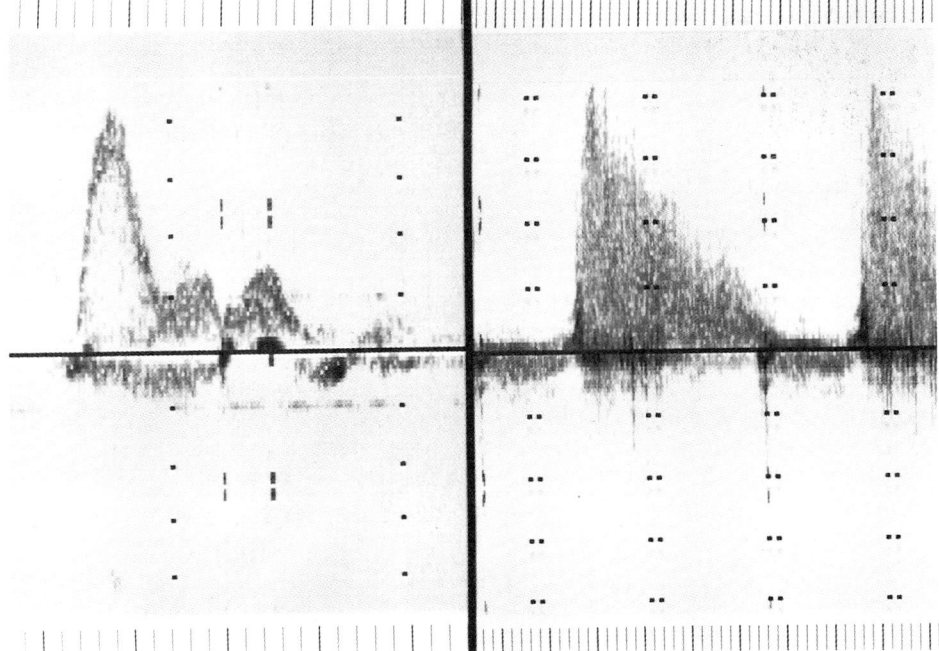

Figure 2.2 Spectral recordings of laminar flow (left) and turbulent flow (right)

vessel area, with the same flow rate through it, therefore tends to make flow become turbulent.

Such a situation may arise when liquid leaves a large tank and enters a relatively small pipe, which is approximately the case of blood leaving one of the ventricles and entering the aorta or pulmonary artery. However, immediately upon entering the pipe, the flow profile is uniform as there has been no chance for viscous friction to act and develop a normal flow profile. Even though the velocity may be high enough to produce turbulent flow, during the initial entry phase it is strictly incorrect to describe it as either laminar or turbulent, and indicators inserted into the stream would show undisturbed flow. The extent of this so called *inlet length* depends on pipe diameter and Reynolds' number. Calculations for the human aorta indicate that the inlet length may be as much as 180 cm, which encompasses all the arterial tree and implies that turbulent flow cannot occur in the cardiovascular system. However, if flow leaving the reservoir is already disturbed, as is the case with the ventricles, the calculation is modified and the inlet length reduces to 10 cm, or somewhere at the top of the aortic arch. Application of this concept to the cardiovascular system is further complicated by pulsatile flow, but it is clear that there is a significant distance, probably at least several centimetres, over which flow remains undisturbed before breaking up and becoming turbulent following a sudden change in vessel diameter, e.g. due to a stenotic ventriculoarterial valve.

Pressure gradients: Bernoulli's theorem

In the eighteenth century, Daniel Bernoulli developed a theory of fluid behaviour, ignoring viscous effects. It is simply a statement of the conservation of energy, applied to two points along a pipe through which fluid is flowing at a constant rate.

If the pipe diameter becomes smaller, the velocity must increase. The kinetic (motion) energy of a unit volume of fluid of density ρ travelling at velocity V1 is equal to $1/2.\rho.V1^2$. After entering the narrower section, its velocity is increased to V2 and the kinetic energy becomes $1/2.\rho.V2^2$. Provided that no energy has been allowed to enter or leave the pipe from outside, the increase in kinetic energy is derived from a fall in its potential energy, which is represented by its pressure. Thus, if the pressures are P1 and P2 respectively, we have the relationship:

$$P1 - P2 = 1/2.\rho.(V2^2 - V1^2)$$

This is known as the Bernoulli equation. It strictly applies only to non-compressible, non-viscous fluids with steady, laminar flow, but the additional terms needed to take account of energy used for viscous friction and acceleration associated with pulsatile flow can usually be ignored.

The application of this equation to derive intracardiac pressure gradients non-invasively from velocity data has largely been responsible for the rapid and widespread introduction of Doppler ultrasound into clinical cardiology. These applications will be dealt with in detail in succeeding chapters, but the principle as applied to mitral stenosis is illustrated in *Figure 2.3*. The upstream chamber is the

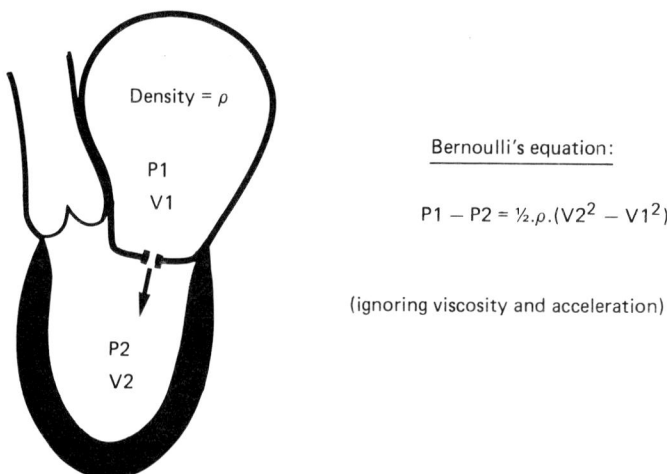

Density = ρ

P1

V1

P2

V2

Bernoulli's equation:

$$P1 - P2 = \tfrac{1}{2}.\rho.(V2^2 - V1^2)$$

(ignoring viscosity and acceleration)

Figure 2.3 Application of Bernoulli's equation to determine the pressure gradient across a stenosed mitral valve. P1, P2 = pressures; V1, V2 = velocities

left atrium, where pressure is relatively high and velocity almost zero. The pressure difference across the diseased mitral valve accelerates the blood and it passes at high velocity into the left ventricle, where the pressure is low. Since the upstream velocity is low, its value squared can be neglected in comparison with the squared value of the jet velocity entering the left ventricle and the Bernoulli equation reduces to:

$$P1 - P2 = 1/2.\rho.V2^2$$

and inserting a value for the density of blood, and measuring the jet velocity in m/s and the pressure gradient in mmHg, this becomes:

$$P1 - P1 = 4.V2^2$$

This simplified equation is adequate for most clinical cardiological applications, but there are occasions where the value of the upstream velocity cannot be ignored, for example when there are two obstructions in series, and then the full expression must be used.

The principle of the Bernoulli equation is the basis of many practical devices, including the aeroplane where increased velocity over the upper, more curved wing surface lowers pressure and provides the lift to raise its mass off the ground.

Further technical considerations

Use of electronic filters

Cardiac structures such as the myocardium and valve leaflets generate very high amplitude signals, but they move relatively slowly. Their Doppler frequencies form high intensity, low frequency artefacts which spoil the appearance of recordings, are unpleasant to listen to on the audio output, and can momentarily paralyse the receiver amplifier causing loss of low intensity signals immediately following them. They can be minimized by using a high-pass filter (i.e. one which allows high frequencies through, but attenuates low frequencies). This removes most of the signals generated by slow moving targets without significantly affecting high Doppler frequencies from blood jets. This filter is often called a *wall motion artefact* or *thump* filter. As the cut-off frequency of the filter is increased, loss of low-frequency components from the Doppler spectrum is evidenced by a widening band around the zero velocity axis on the display (*Figure 2.4*). To determine a

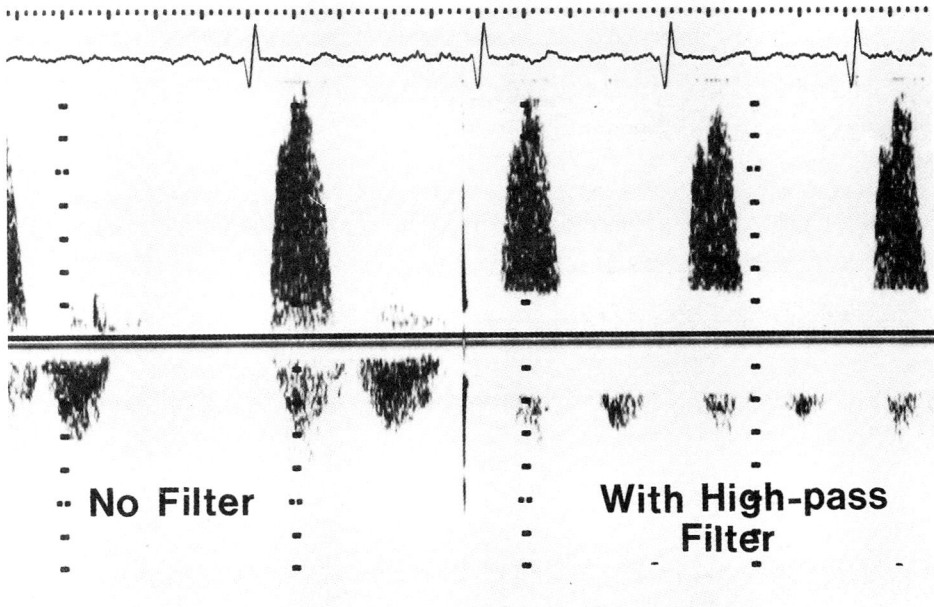

Figure 2.4 Spectral recording of flow in the ascending aorta, showing the effect of increasing the cut-off frequency of the high-pass filter

pressure gradient using the Bernoulli equation, it is necessary to show clearly the highest velocity present in a blood jet. This generates the highest Doppler frequency but its amplitude can be low and it may be submerged in the electronic noise present in the recording system. Filters are therefore usually provided to enhance the high Doppler frequencies and to separate them from still higher frequency electronic noise. Optimizing these filters represents one of the major elements of skill in equipment design.

Part of the technology of improving Doppler signal-to-noise ratio involves providing a degree of automatic gain control (AGC). This technique is widely used, e.g. in dictating machines, to control the level of amplification according to the intensity of the input signal. In the absence of any input, the machine increases the amplification level until the electronic hiss of the amplifier is heard. This can sometimes cause confusion in Doppler, e.g. when studying a patient who has aortic stenosis and may have additional mild aortic regurgitation. The intense signal from the stenotic jet requires relatively little amplification and so the background signals are not evident but, during diastole, with little or no input signal, the amplifier increases its gain to maximum and then a faint high frequency signal, which mimics aortic regurgitation but actually is artefact, is heard and recorded.

Audio outputs

By chance, the Doppler shift generated by blood at velocities encountered in the cardiovascular system (1–5 m/s) and at ultrasound frequencies of 2–3 MHz is in the range of 3–10 kHz, frequencies which are well within the range of the human ear.

It is, therefore, a simple matter to present the Doppler frequencies as an audible signal, sometimes in stereo with flow towards the transducer fed to one channel and flow away from it to the other. The velocity is represented by the pitch of the sound. Laminar flow is indicated by pure whistling tones and turbulence by much harsher noises. By harnessing the excellent tonal recognition qualities of the ear, the experienced operator can both assess the presence of abnormal flow patterns and ensure that the signal quality is good and free from artefact. Indeed this often indicates that the Doppler beam is near the desired flow area before its demonstration on the spectrum analyser and, in some machines, although a low intensity signal may just be audible, the spectrum analyser may be unable to display it.

Integration of imaging and Doppler

Using pulsed wave Doppler, it is possible to record simultaneously an M-mode echocardiogram on which the depth of the Doppler gate can be shown, together with a spectral velocity plot. It is also possible with electronically steered (phased array) two-dimensional scanners to record simultaneously M-mode and two-dimensional images. However, this necessitates using most of the available ultrasound pulses to form the two-dimensional image, with only about 500/s assigned to the M-mode. This lowers the Nyquist limit to 250 Hz and, although a very crude audible and visual indication of flow may be possible, it is of no practical use for Doppler analysis. Therefore, in practice, the machine, whether a mechanical or phased array scanner, forms a two-dimensional image and then freezes this while transmitting all pulses in the direction required for Doppler. The two-dimensional image is up-dated at intervals, which can be varied by the operator from every 1 to 20 seconds typically and synchronized with the ECG if desired, during which period the spectral display is momentarily turned off.

With continuous wave there is no possibility of obtaining even an M-mode image simultaneously. Some manufacturers offer transducers which combine multi-element phased-array imaging crystals with two additional crystals for continuous wave Doppler. This avoids the operator needing to change transducers when switching from imaging to Doppler, but the combined transducer is generally larger and more difficult to position over a restricted acoustic window on the patient's chest, since the axis of the imaging elements is not the same as that of the Doppler crystals. This problem can be overcome in mechanically scanned transducers which combine imaging and Doppler functions in a single crystal which has a relatively small contact area on the chest. Another difficulty arises because transducers for imaging use much mechanical damping to prevent the crystals vibrating after they are pulsed, whereas for continuous wave Doppler high damping is undesirable. Thus the potential advantage of having imaging and Doppler in the same transducer tends to be offset in practice by a larger, more expensive and less sensitive transducer.

Sample volume length in pulsed wave Doppler

Almost all machines allow the operator to vary the length of the sample volume in the pulsed wave mode. If the gate is set to its minimum length, usually about 2 mm, more precise location of a flow pattern is possible. However, at a frequency of 2 MHz the sample length corresponds to only three ultrasound wavelengths. The Fourier spectrum of a short pulse of waves of a single frequency contains many additional harmonics and introduces uncertainty into the spectral analysis of the received echoes. On the other hand, as the length of the sample gate is increased, there is increasing uncertainty about the location of the flow detected. At the extreme, in the continuous wave mode the sample gate is effectively infinite and there is no depth information at all. In practice, use of a sample gate length less than 5 mm is not recommended unless there is a need for very precise location of flow and for most applications a gate length of more than 10 mm is not required.

Choice of ultrasound frequency for Doppler

For imaging, the highest possible ultrasound frequency is used consistent with obtaining a strong enough echo to form an image free of excessive electronic noise. For Doppler, there are advantages to be gained from using a low frequency. First, in the pulsed wave mode, the aliasing frequency is directly proportional to the transmitted frequency: at the same working depth, halving the ultrasound frequency, e.g. from 5 MHz to 2.5 MHz doubles the maximum velocity that can be recorded without aliasing. Another reason for preferring a low frequency is that attenuation of ultrasound is much less and relatively stronger echoes are received. At 2 MHz, 50% attenuation occurs for every 2 cm of beam length, whereas at 5 MHz the same attenuation occurs in only 1 cm. This difference may not seem too important, but at a working depth of 10 cm, for which the total path length is 20 cm, the relative attenuation factors are $(1/2)^{10}$ and $(1/2)^{20}$ respectively, i.e. the echo strength at 5 MHz is only 1/1024 of that at 2 MHz.

Finally, for many applications, the relatively wider ultrasound beam at a lower frequency is actually an advantage. To apply the Bernoulli equation it is necessary to detect the *highest* jet velocity present. Jets through stenosed valves can be eccentric and a narrow beam can fail to detect the maximum velocity, whereas a wider beam will encompass it. The ultrasound frequency currently favoured for continuous wave Doppler is in the range 1.5–2 MHz.

Compensation for incorrect beam alignment

As discussed earlier, if the ultrasound beam is not perfectly aligned with the direction of blood flow, the velocity measured is lower than the true value by a factor of (cosine θ), where θ is the angle between flow axis and ultrasound beam. Bearing in mind that when using the Bernoulli equation pressure gradients are derived from the squares of the velocities, significant errors can be introduced by incorrect beam/jet alignment. For example, if the measured velocity is 4 m/s, equivalent to a pressure gradient of 64 mmHg, but there is an angle error of 30°, the true velocity should have been $4/\cos 30° = 4.62$ m/s, which corresponds to a pressure gradient of 85 mmHg, a 25% underestimation.

Most machines provide a facility for applying the angle cosine correction. A second cursor is rotated until it is aligned with the flow, as assessed from inspection of the two-dimensional image. The cosine of the angle between this and the main M-mode cursor is then calculated automatically and used to re-scale the velocity calibration on the recording. Provided that the second cursor can be perfectly aligned with the direction of flow, this method provides the required correction but, in practice, we are dealing with a three-dimensional system and the two-dimensional image does not provide any information about the angle between the blood flow and the ultrasound beam in the elevation plane, at right angles to that of the scan. It is thus almost always the case that there will be a residual angle error. Suppose this is ± 10°. If, by manipulating the transducer, the beam and flow are thought to be aligned, the actual angle between the two is 0 ± 10°. The cosine correction is nominally zero and actually 0.984 which, when squared, gives a pressure gradient error of 3%. If, however, the nominal angle is 30° and the angle corrector is used to compensate for this, but there is the *same* error of ± 10°, the cosine corrections of 20° and 40° are 0.939 and 0.766, compared with the actual correction applied of 0.866. When squared, the resulting pressure gradient error is +22% or −17%. This is illustrated geometrically in *Figure 2.5*. The angle corrector tends to give a false impression of accuracy and the reader is strongly advised not to use it, but instead to try always to achieve correct alignment of the beam and blood flow. If this cannot be achieved, it is probably best to accept that the velocity measured is lower than the true value, and not to attempt quantitative correction. Colour Doppler, by demonstrating the direction of a jet may give the impression that angle correction can be undertaken with greater accuracy, but the potential for multiplying any error in angle measurement is unchanged.

Extended range or high pulse repetition frequency Doppler

Extended range, or high pulse repetition frequency (PRF) Doppler is an ingenious way of partly overcoming the limitation imposed by aliasing on the measurement of high blood velocities by pulsed wave Doppler. To understand how it works, consider measurement of velocity through the mitral valve from an apical transducer position as shown in *Figure 2.6a*. Using normal pulsed wave Doppler the sample volume is positioned in the mitral orifice. Echoes returning after a time

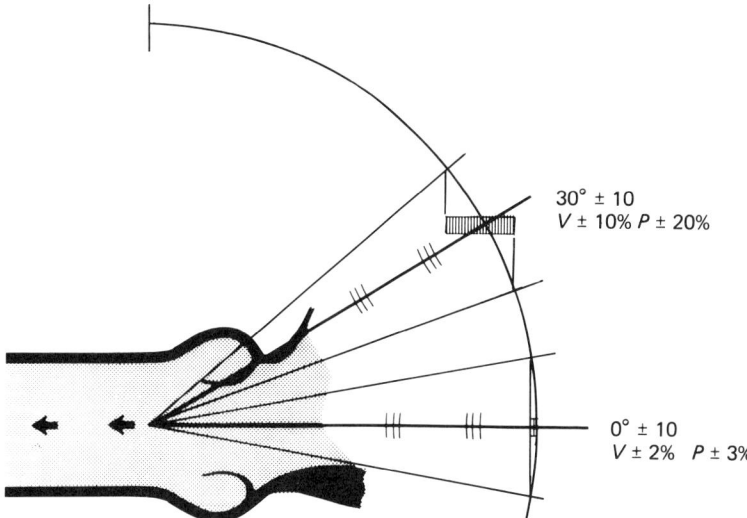

30° ± 10
V ± 10% P ± 20%

0° ± 10
V ± 2% P ± 3%

Figure 2.5 Diagram showing the errors in velocity and pressure calculations caused by incorrect alignment of the ultrasound beam and blood flow. The same error of ± 10° has much greater effect when the nominal angle is 30° than when it is 0°

delay appropriate to this range are analysed to provide both structural information about the mitral valve and information on velocity through it. A second pulse can be sent immediately after these echoes have returned. The pulse rate is limited by the range of the mitral valve from the transducer and the maximum measurable velocity can be calculated from the range × velocity product for the ultrasound frequency being used.

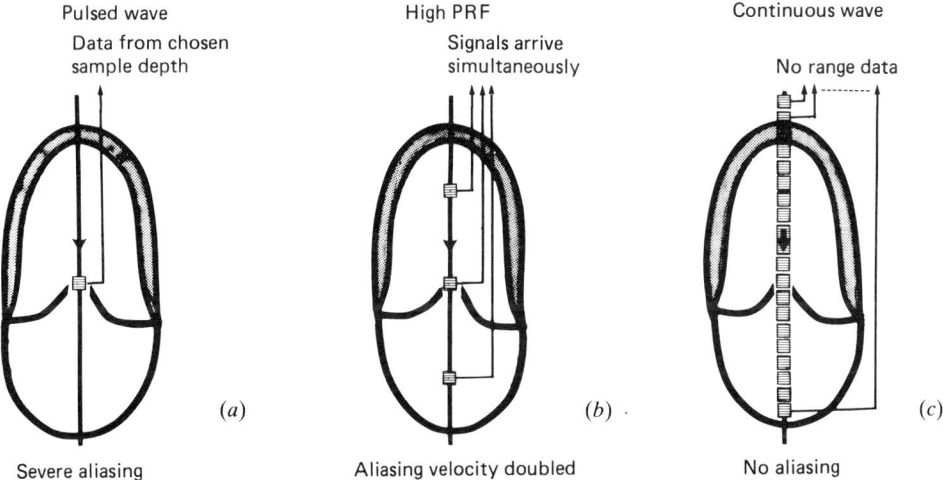

Pulsed wave
Data from chosen
sample depth

High PRF
Signals arrive
simultaneously

Continuous wave

No range data

(a)   (b)   (c)

Severe aliasing   Aliasing velocity doubled   No aliasing

Figure 2.6 Diagram showing the principle of high PRF Doppler. Increasing the pulse frequency offers a compromise between the features of pulsed and continuous wave systems

If the pulse rate is doubled, at the moment when an echo from a particular pulse returns to the transducer from the mitral valve, an echo from the next pulse arrives back from a point halfway between the transducer and the valve. It, too, contains both structural and velocity information, which is superimposed on that obtained from the first pulse in the mitral orifice. In effect two Doppler sample volumes are in use simultaneously, as shown in *Figure 2.6b*. This could be very confusing but by careful choice of beam direction it is usually possible to ensure that velocity and structural data from the proximal sample are of relatively little importance, as in the example where it is in the middle of the left ventricular cavity. The advantage that this technique offers is that the total number of pulses passing through the mitral valve orifice is doubled, and therefore the aliasing velocity is doubled.

Further extension by quadrupling the pulse rate is possible. It can be seen that increasing the PRF improves the quantification of velocity data, but at the expense of introducing ambiguity in the spatial data. Taken to its extreme, if the number of pulses transmitted is increased to the point where the pulses merge together all spatial data are lost, but there is now no problem with aliasing and we have returned to continuous wave operation (*Figure 2.6c*). High PRF Doppler thus offers a compromise between continuous wave and pulsed wave. It shares both the advantages and disadvantages of each method.

3

The normal Doppler examination and flow patterns

Neil Wilson

It is often possible to recognize obvious or gross examples of pathology without being confident in the recognition of all aspects of normality. However, with Doppler ultrasound it is important that the normal patterns are known as the technique can have particular application in allowing the distinction to be made between patients with mild cardiac disease and subjects with a completely normal heart. It is recommended that the operator establishes a flexible routine for Doppler examination during an echocardiographic study with the aim of making a comprehensive study of blood velocity across all four cardiac valves and in the great arteries and veins, thus ensuring that conclusions are drawn on the full findings and not on the basis of a single velocity recording. The following description should form the basis for the reader to adjust and develop his or her own style of performing a Doppler examination. Small practical points will be outlined which could be thought to be unconventional but which have been developed as a result of experience in obtaining certain velocity patterns. If a non-imaging transducer is used considerable practice may be required to obtain the signals. Most duplex scanners have steerable pulsed Doppler, but some do not have a steerable continuous wave beam and others do not even have on-line continuous wave Doppler. Thus the use of pulsed and continuous wave Doppler may demand different techniques and for each operator the exact technique will depend on the equipment used.

There are few references to normal peak velocities in the heart and great vessels. Some studies[1, 2] concentrated on important single site measurements such as the aorta. Later published data have included intracardiac sites[3, 4, 5] as Doppler interrogation of these positions increased in clinical awareness and importance.

Systematic Doppler examination

The position and comfort of the patient are often taken for granted but are important for obtaining a satisfactory Doppler study which may take some time to perform and requires that the patient keeps still. The examination requires concentration, patience and dexterity on behalf of the examiner, so he or she should also be comfortable; some operators like to stand to conduct the study but others prefer high stools. The study can be performed from either side of the patient and that used for echocardiography should be used since Doppler examination is really only an extension of this.

Patient positioning is approximately the same as for a two-dimensional echocardiographic study with most signals obtained with the patient supine with the trunk supported at 30–45° to the body. Lateral decubitus positions are frequently employed, the left particularly to study the right ventricular outflow tract and the right for interrogating the ascending aorta. With experience it is possible to record Doppler signals from most sites in the majority of subjects but, of course, obese or emphysematous patients or those with a chest deformity may defeat the most experienced examiner.

Children are less of a problem for imaging, although lack of cooperation on their part may cause considerable difficulty. Although satisfactory echocardiographic images can often be obtained from a moving child, good quality Doppler records require the patient to be stationary for more than a second or two at a time. Failing the usual reassuring routines with explanation, toys, and the presence of parents, it is sometimes necessary to sedate infants and toddlers to obtain a complete study; this measure is easily justified by the additional valuable information obtained.

It must be constantly borne in mind that the best quality velocity signals are obtained when the sample volume of the Doppler beam is parallel to the direction of flow and thus transducer positions are often different from those used for imaging. When using two-dimensional echocardiography with pulsed Doppler, it is very tempting to look at the two-dimensional image and assume that a sample volume placed midway between the walls of an artery or between the leaflets of a valve will automatically detect the maximum velocity. It is essential to remember the very important principle in the use of Doppler, that flow is in three dimensions and the two-dimensional image serves only as a guide within which further small adjustments of the transducer and sample volume must be made in order to record the best Doppler signals. At all times care must be taken to ensure that the spectral signal shows a well defined maximum velocity envelope and that the audio signal is as close as possible to a pure tone, which sounds rather like a hiss or a high-pitched whistle when the sample beam is correctly aligned with flow. Thus for each recording position fine adjustment of the angulation is made independent of the two-dimensional image.

In practice, if an imaging transducer is used, it is usual to perform the Doppler and echocardiographic study simultaneously, thus obtaining the echocardiographic information and velocity measurements at the same time as the examination proceeds. To perform separate M-mode, two-dimensional and Doppler studies would be rather rigid and can be time consuming. However, some clinicians prefer this and it is necessary if a non-imaging transducer is used; continuous wave studies can usually be obtained fairly easily but pulsed ones[6] take considerable time to perform and experience to learn. The recording may, nevertheless, be better than that obtained with an imaging system where there is a danger that insufficient attention is paid to the audio and spectral signals to obtain the optimal one. Even when using an imaging system it may be better to use continuous wave to obtain the clearest signal and then switch to pulsed wave to localize it.

By convention, blood flow towards the transducer is displayed by a time velocity waveform above the zero or base line (positive deflection) while flow away from it is displayed as a time velocity waveform below the zero line (negative deflection). An electrocardiogram (ECG) should always be displayed with the spectral tracing to assist in timing the cardiac events.

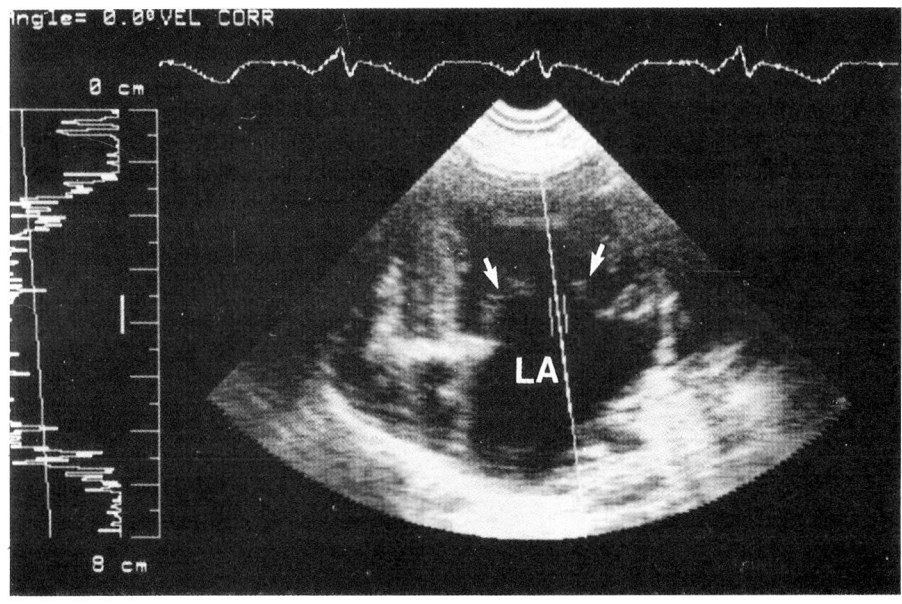

(a)

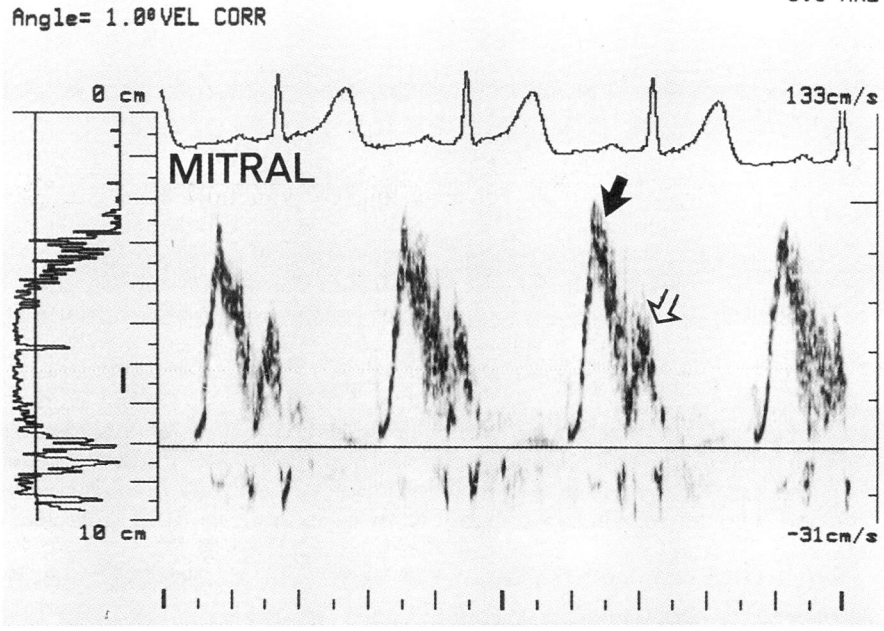

(b)

Figure 3.1 Recording of the mitral time velocity waveform. (a) The sample volume (parallel lines) is astride the cursor line midway between the open mitral valve leaflets (arrowed). (b) The early velocity peak (solid arrow) is due to passive ventricular filling (E wave) and is followed by the smaller velocity peak (open arrow) due to atrial contraction (A wave). LA, left atrium

Mitral valve

With pulsed Doppler echocardiography and a duplex scanner, mitral valve flow velocities are best obtained by using an apical four chamber view which is tilted towards the axilla to bring the ventricular septum almost vertical (*Figure 3.1a*) and then placing the sample volume midway between the leaflets of the mitral valve. The characteristic waveform is M-shaped and mimics that of the M-mode recording of the mitral valve. The two components of the wave form, denoted the E and A wave (*Figure 3.1b*), are due to passive ventricular filling and atrial contraction respectively. Under normal circumstances, in both adults and children, the E wave velocity is considerably higher than the A. The range of the E wave velocity[5] is 44–128 cm/s with a mean of 77 cm/s (*Table 3.1*). Variation in the configuration of

Table 3.1 Normal peak velocity in the heart and great vessels

Site	Range (cm/s)	Mean (cm/s)	1 standard deviation
Superior vena cava	28–80	51	13
Tricuspid valve	33–81	53	12
Pulmonary artery	52–131	81	17
Mitral valve	44–128	77	16
Ascending aorta	76–155	104	19
Descending aorta	70–160	101	17

the mitral velocity occurs with fast heart rates and atrial fibrillation. In tachycardia the A wave is not identified because of fusion with the E wave, while in atrial fibrillation clearly there can be no recognizable A wave and the E wave velocity varies from beat to beat. With a non-imaging transducer mitral valve flow is most easily recorded with continuous wave Doppler by placing the transducer close to the cardiac apex and steering the beam posteriorly and towards the left manubriosternal joint. The characteristic M-shaped wave form is not as pronounced as with the pulsed study, due to the different spectral signal obtained. Occasionally the beam will abut on to the left ventricular outflow tract and flow through it will appear as negatively directed velocities on the same display as the mitral flow. Pulsed Doppler can then be used to record flow at specific levels, although it takes some practice to become adept at this.

Tricuspid valve

With pulsed Doppler and two-dimensional imaging the tricuspid valve flow velocity is best obtained by using a slightly foreshortened apical or subcostal four chamber view with the sample volume placed midway between the leaflets of the open tricuspid valve (*Figure 3.2a* and *b*). Once again small adjustments of transducer angle are often necessary to maximize the signal velocity. The tricuspid waveform is very variable: it may be considered as being M-shaped with the E and A waves of passive ventricular filling and atrial contraction, but close inspection demonstrates that there are three components to this wave form[7]. In normal circumstances the E wave velocity is greater than the A wave, although often the two cannot be separated, particularly with tachycardia and atrial arrhythmias. Peak E wave velocities range from 33 to 81 cm/s with a mean of 53 cm/s (*see Table 3.1*). With a non-imaging transducer, continuous wave interrogation of tricuspid velocities is

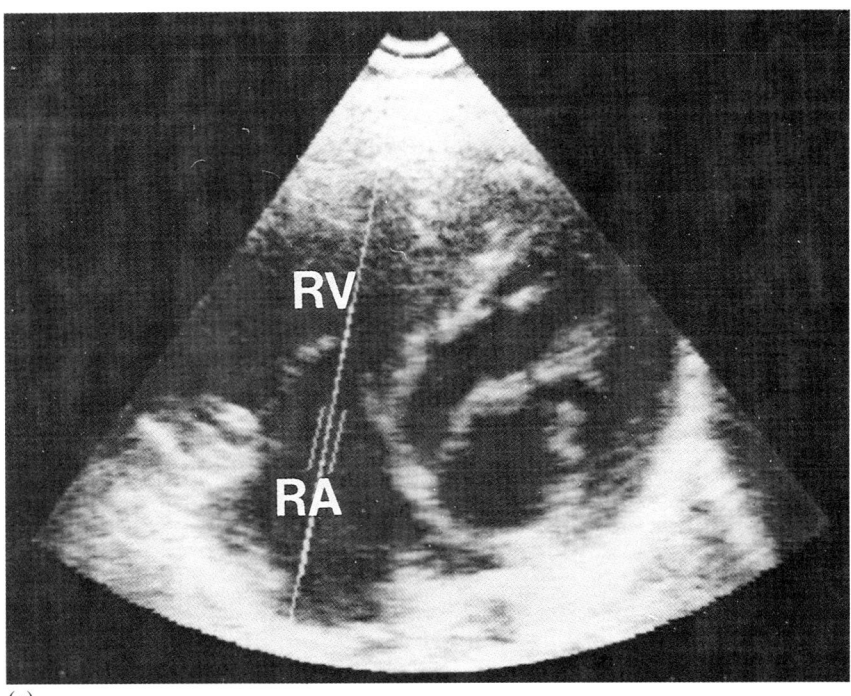

(a)

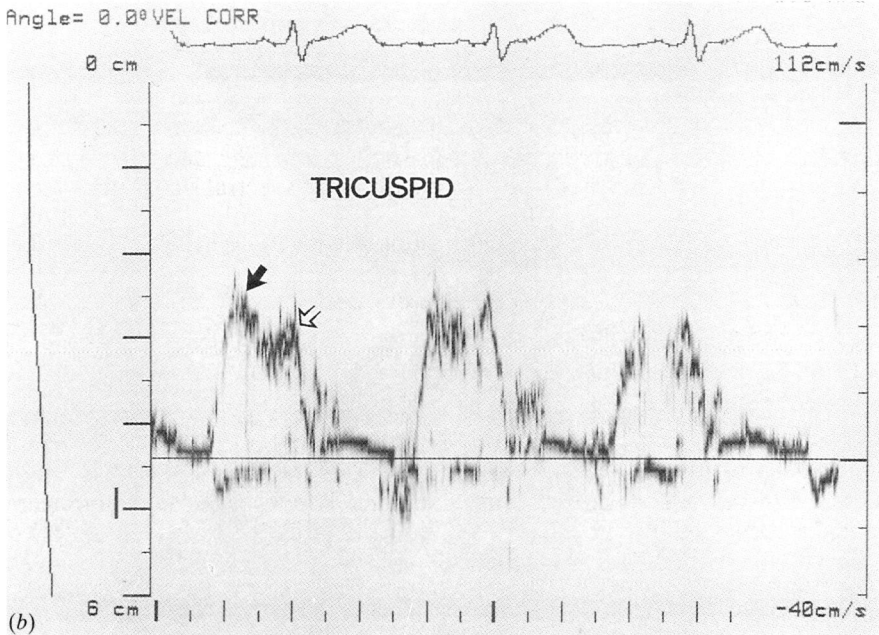

(b)

Figure 3.2 Recording of the tricuspid time velocity waveform. (*a*) The sample volume is between the leaflets of the tricuspid valve. (*b*) The early velocity peak (solid arrow) is due to passive ventricular filling (E wave) and is followed by the smaller velocity peak (open arrow) due to atrial contraction (A wave). RA, right atrium; RV, right ventricle

best obtained from the lower left sternal edge with a transducer aimed posteriorly and to the patient's right. In older children and adults it is not unusual to obtain not only the positive velocities of diastolic flow but also a fleeting high velocity systolic signal directed away from the transducer, representing a degree of tricuspid regurgitation, which may be a completely normal finding as discussed in Chapter 6. Tricuspid flow may be distinguished from mitral by the fact that the maximum velocity is generally lower and varies with respiration.

Pulmonary artery

Pulmonary artery flow velocities are often best obtained from the left parasternal short axis transducer position. With imaging, the sample volume is placed in the main pulmonary artery midway between the pulmonary valve and bifurcation (*Figure 3.3a*). The signal can also be obtained from the subxiphoid position and this is particularly important in patients with valve abnormalities. A single systolic peak travelling away from the transducer is obtained, its peak ranging from 52 to 131 cm/s with a mean of 81 cm/s (*Figure 3.3b*). In addition, if the wall filter is set sufficiently low it may be possible to demonstrate a short low velocity late diastolic peak of 20 cm/s or less representing antegrade blood flow caused by atrial contraction[7] similar to the A wave on M-mode echocardiography.

Aorta

The aortic valve flow velocity may be obtained from many transducer positions, the conventional ones being the suprasternal notch, right supraclavicular fossa, high right sternal edge and the subxiphoid, subcostal, and apical sites. The two most frequently used are the apex and suprasternal notch. From the apex, the left ventricular outflow tract, aortic valve, and ascending aorta are imaged in a five chamber view displaying mitral and aortic valve continuity; the sample volume can then be moved progressively from the outflow tract through the aortic valve to the proximal ascending aorta to measure the velocities at each site. To obtain signals from the suprasternal notch the patient's neck is extended by placing a pillow beneath the shoulders and the transducer positioned in the notch; for optimal signals the transducer may have to be placed quite deeply and this can be uncomfortable.

With an in-line imaging transducer it is difficult to obtain a complete image of both walls of the ascending aorta and it may only be possible to place the sample volume within 20 or 30° to the axis of the actual flow. This problem can be surmounted by using an imaging system with a steerable or off-line Doppler beam which can show the valve and both walls of the ascending aorta simultaneously and allow appropriate positioning of the pulsed sample volume. On the other hand, non-imaging transducers, such as the early continuous wave type, are often made with an angle in the head which facilitates the measurement of aortic velocity from the suprasternal notch. The transducer is placed in the notch and angled downwards and slightly to the left and tilted anteriorly until the optimal signal is obtained. From the apex the velocity waveform shows a negative deflection (*Figure 3.4a*) and obviously from the suprasternal notch it is positive (*Figure 3.4b*); the peak velocity is 76–155 cm/s with a mean of 104 cm/s.

Because of the eccentricity of some stenotic jets it is useful to measure the aortic valve velocities from other sites in patients with aortic valve disease. The size and

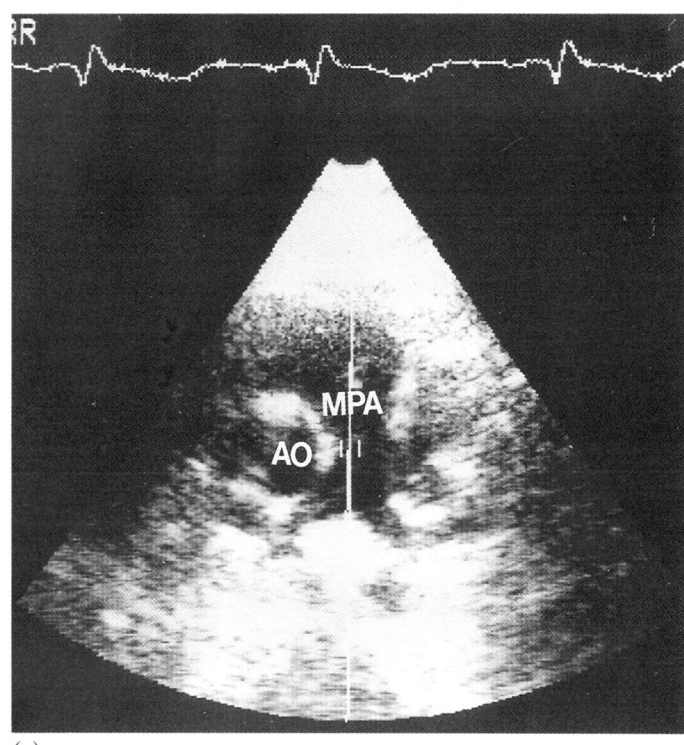

(a)

3.5 MHz

Angle= 1.0⁰VEL CORR

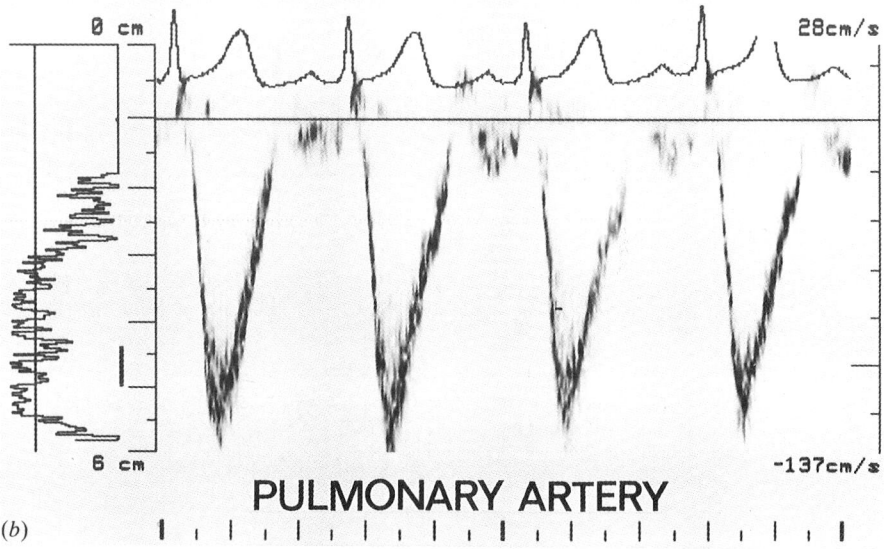

PULMONARY ARTERY

(b)

Figure 3.3 Recording of the pulmonary time velocity waveform. (*a*) The sample volume is in the main pulmonary artery viewed from the left parasternal short axis position. (*b*) There is a single systolic peak followed by a lower velocity diastolic one. MPA, main pulmonary artery; AO, aorta

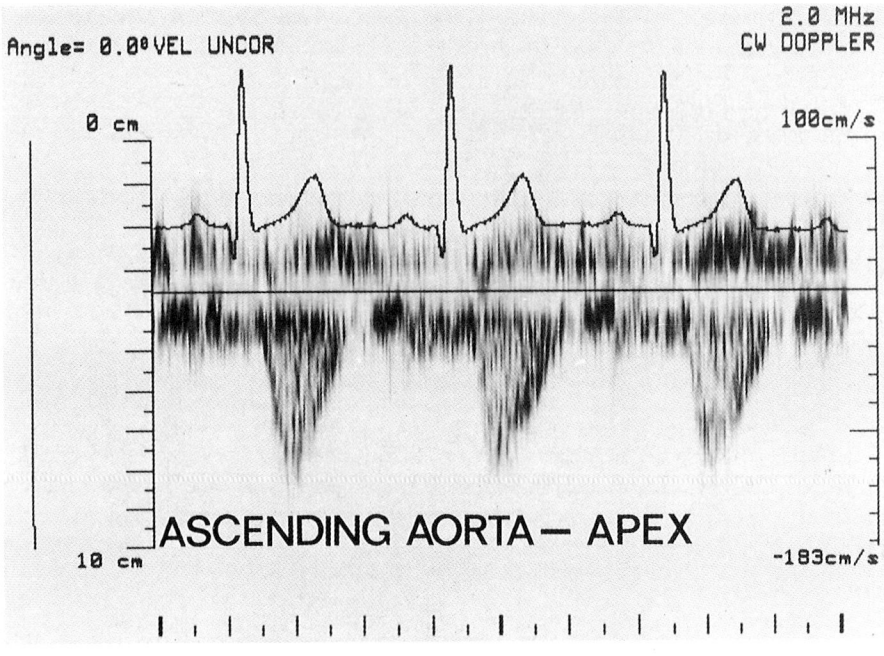

(a)

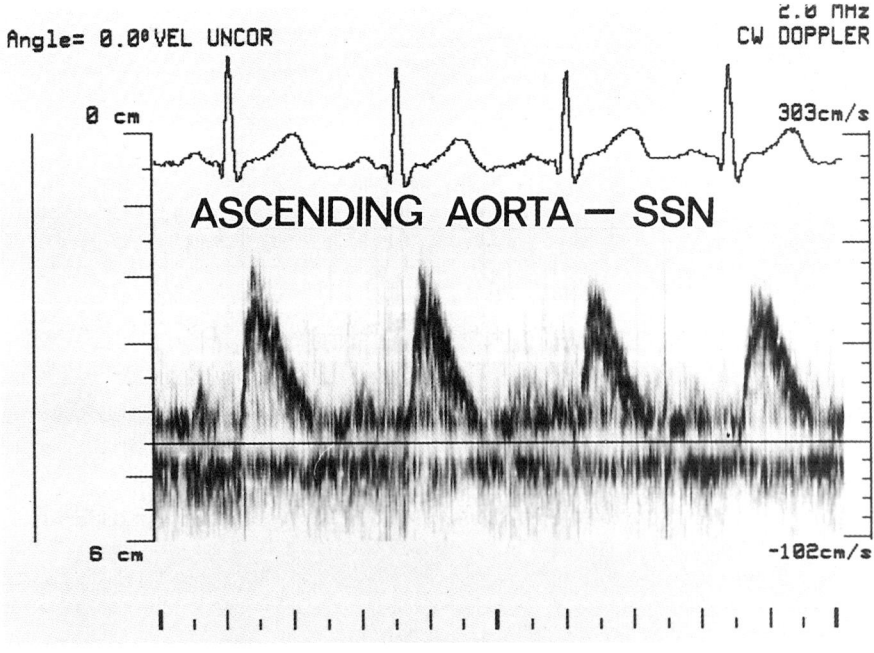

(b)

Figure 3.4 Time velocity waveform of ascending aortic blood flow obtained from (*a*) the apex and (*b*) the suprasternal notch, using a continuous wave transducer. There is a single systolic peak directed away from the transducer from the apex and towards it from the suprasternal notch. SSN, suprasternal notch

shape of most imaging transducers make their use difficult in this context. The small size of the non-imaging ones uniquely suits them to obtain these aortic signals since very precise positioning and angulation is often required. These transducers are most often used for continuous wave Doppler recordings.

From the apex, the transducer is placed in a very similar position to that for mitral velocities, but is tilted slightly more anteriorly and towards the right manubriosternal joint. It usually fits quite snugly into the suprasternal notch and may be directed downwards and slightly to the left and anteriorly to obtain the maximum velocity. From the right upper sternal edge, at approximately the second intercostal space, the transducer is directed downwards towards the apex and slightly posteriorly. Signals are often best obtained from here with the patient in the right lateral decubitus position. The present author finds the right supraclavicular fossa difficult to use but it is essential in cases of aortic stenosis where it may give the maximum jet velocity. From this site, the transducer is tilted downwards and slightly to the left aiming approximately for the apex. With eccentric jets, aortic velocity may best be measured from the subcostal or subxiphoid positions by tilting the transducer up towards the upper left sternal edge.

Descending aorta

Descending aortic velocities can be measured easily by imaging the aortic arch from either the suprasternal notch or high parasternal position. With pulsed wave Doppler, the sample volume is placed just distal to the left subclavian artery (*Figure 3.5a*). The velocity waveform is displayed away from the transducer and typical velocity values of 70–160 cm/s, mean 101 cm/s, are obtained (*Figure 3.5b*). With non-imaging Doppler the transducer is placed in the suprasternal notch and directed posteriorly downwards and to the left. It is important to note that descending aortic velocities can approach 2.0 m/s and care must be taken not to diagnose stenotic lesions such as coarctation of the aorta without obtaining proximal velocities and demonstrating that they are considerably lower. The change in direction and effect of gravity on blood flowing around the arch and into the head and neck vessels produces relative turbulence, increasing modal peak velocity of the red cells in this area. In addition, it is not unusual to detect low velocity diastolic blood flow directed towards the transducer from the descending aorta (*Figure 3.5b*). The exact cause of this is not known, but it probably represents the combined effect of elastic recoil of the aorta and filling of the sinuses of Valsalva and coronary arteries in diastole.

Superior vena cava

The superior vena cava flow may be recorded from the suprasternal notch with imaging, with the sample volume placed parallel to the aorta (*Figure 3.6a*) or from its junction with the right atrium from the subcostal region by tilting the transducer up towards the right sternal edge. The velocity recording is biphasic with systolic and diastolic peaks of which the systolic is usually the greater (*Figure 3.6b*). From the suprasternal notch the waveforms are displayed away from the transducer and from the subcostal approach towards it, i.e. above the zero line. Peak velocities are approximately equal from either site and in the region of 28–80 cm/s with a mean of 51 cm/s and can vary with respiration. The phasic nature of this and other venous waveforms is frequently disturbed by obstructed breathing, crying, the Valsalva manoeuvre and pericardial or right heart pathology.

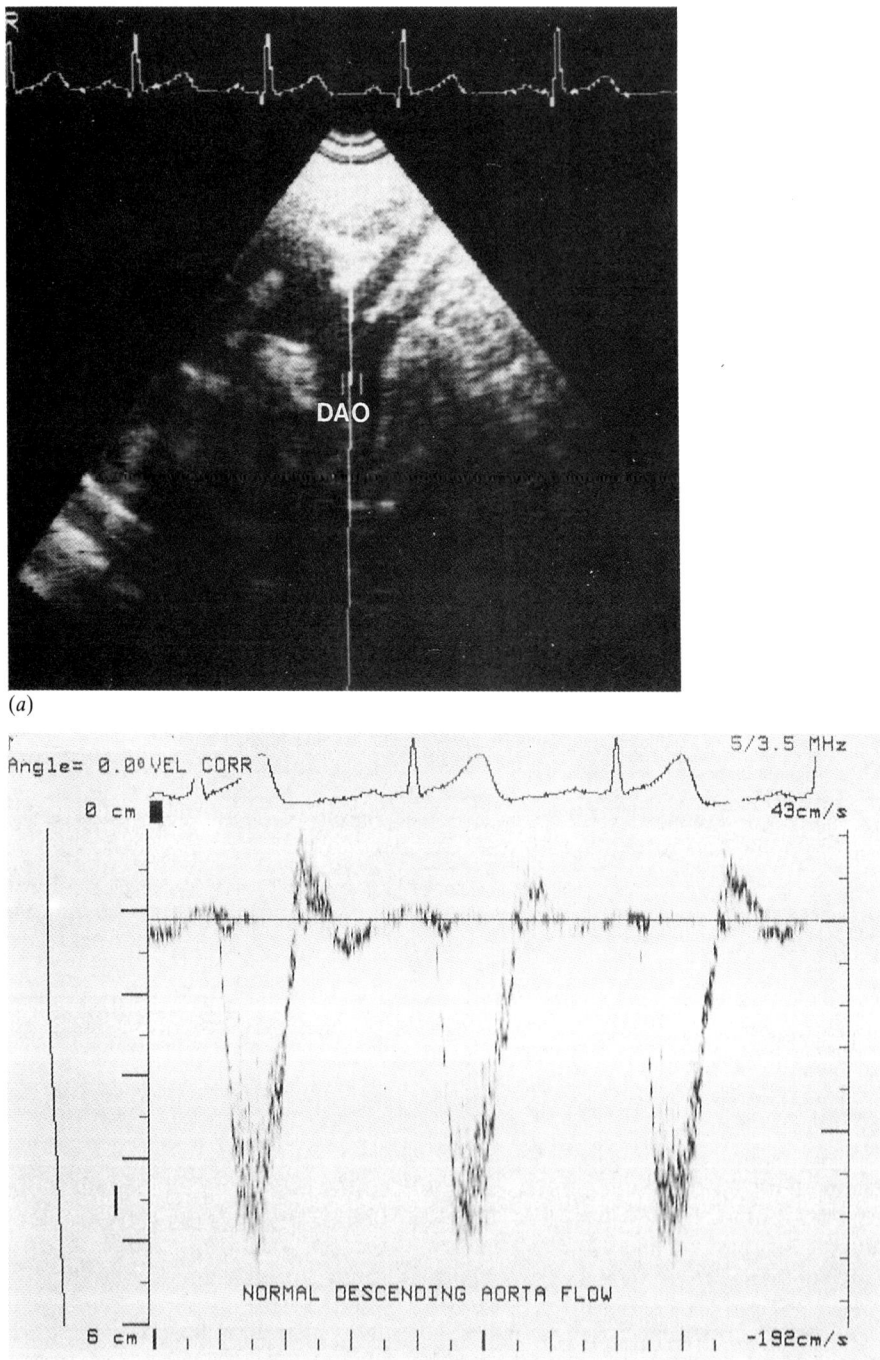

(a)

(b)

Figure 3.5 Recording of the time velocity waveform of descending aortic blood flow. (a) The sample volume in descending aorta imaged from the suprasternal notch. (b) There is a single systolic peak followed by a low velocity peak in the opposite direction in diastole. DAO, descending aorta

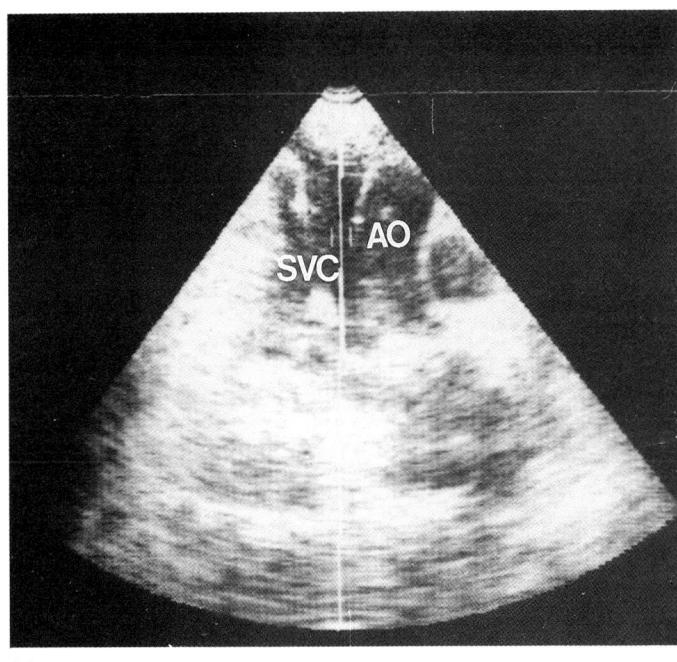

(a)

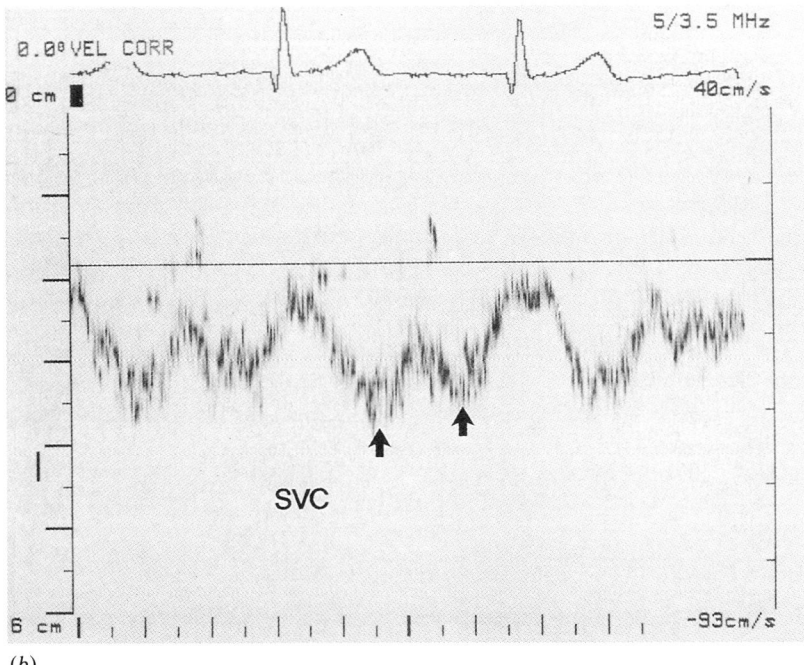

(b)

Figure 3.6 Recording of the time velocity waveform of superior vena caval flow. (*a*) The sample volume is in the superior vena cava in close proximity to the aorta. (*b*) The waveform has systolic and diastolic peaks. AO, aorta; SVC, superior vena cava

Measurement of superior vena cava velocities can be of clinical value in abnormalities of venous return such as a cerebral arteriovenous malformation or total anomalous pulmonary venous return, and in postoperative assessment following intra-atrial surgery such as the Mustard or Senning procedure for transposition of the great arteries. In addition, pathological tricuspid regurgitation will produce significant positive velocity recordings when the superior vena cava flow is recorded from the suprasternal notch.

With a non-imaging transducer, recordings of superior vena cava velocity are best made in the continuous wave mode and can be obtained again from either the suprasternal or subcostal position by directing the transducer in a similar way as for duplex studies.

Time to peak velocity in the pulmonary artery

This measurement has been shown by several workers[8] to be a rough guide to pulmonary artery pressure. The measurement is described as the time taken for the velocity wave form recorded in the pulmonary artery to depart the base line and reach modal peak velocity. The time to peak velocity ranges between 60 and 180 ms with a mean of 120 ms. In older children and adults, a time to peak velocity of less than 90 ms has been shown almost invariably to be associated with pulmonary hypertension. The correlation is inverse and although quite strong, with r values approximately 0.8, the standard error of this estimate is very large precluding it as an individual predictor of pulmonary pressure in any individual.

Changes of peak velocity with age and body surface area

In general there is a weak inverse correlation between peak velocity and body surface area and age, with typical r values ranging from 0.2 for the tricuspid valve to 0.53 for the superior vena cava[5]. Although it can be considered statistically significant, the correlation is weak and has little practical implication. In the present author's study of children and young adults, ascending and descending

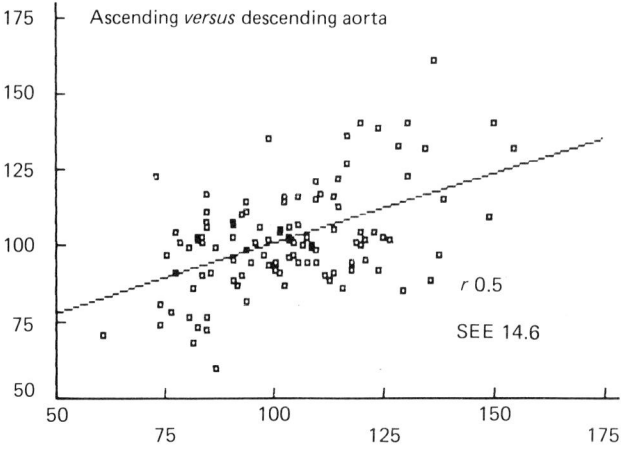

Figure 3.7 Correlation between ascending (horizontal axis) and descending aortic velocity in the same subject (units cm/s). There is significant correlation, but the scatter is too wide to allow substitution in the volumetric flow calculation for cardiac output (*see* text). r, correlation coefficient; SEE, standard error of the estimate

aortic velocities did not change significantly with age or body surface area, but another study of patients aged up to 80 years old[2] demonstrated a decline in maximal aortic velocity with age. The time to peak velocity in the pulmonary artery does lengthen significantly with age.

Correlation of peak velocity at different sites in the same individual is very weak and, in practical terms, does not permit the substitution of velocity at one site to be used in the volumetric flow calculation for cardiac output at another. Some workers have advocated using an ascending aortic cross-sectional area with a descending aortic mean velocity to calculate cardiac output. *Figure 3.7* demonstrates the correlation between ascending and descending aortic velocity in the same subject. It can be seen that although the *r* value is signficant at a high level ($P \leqslant 0.01$), the standard error is far too wide to allow substitution of values.

Variations of normality which may be misconstrued as abnormal

Atrioventricular valve velocity

Variations in the configuration of the mitral and tricuspid velocities occur commonly with fast heart rates when there is fusion of the E and A waves. In addition, in dysrhythmias the A wave may be lost completely, as in atrial fibrillation, or may bear an abnormal time relation to the E wave, as in complete heart block. Because of the proximity of the left ventricular outflow tract to mitral inflow, the incorporation of its flow velocity with the mitral when using a non-imaging continuous wave transducer may give the impression of mitral regurgitation to the untrained observer; however, unless there is aortic stenosis the maximum velocity from the aorta will be much less than that from mitral regurgitation. Clearly, when analysing wave forms at different sites, proximity of other structures must constantly be borne in mind, especially when using continuous wave Doppler as velocities throughout the beam will be recorded whether purposely or not. The dominance of the E wave in the mitral and tricuspid wave form is often reversed in the face of a poorly compliant ventricle or with elevated ventricular end diastolic pressure[9] leading to a higher velocity peak from atrial contraction.

Peak velocity at all sites may be increased in the absence of stenosis by increased volumetric blood flow across that site, most commonly found in children with a left to right shunt. In a study of increased blood velocities in the heart and great vessels in congenital heart disease[10], approximately 80% of patients had increased blood velocity across one or more normal valves. For example, children with an atrial septal defect are likely to have increased tricuspid and pulmonary artery velocities. These velocity increases are relatively modest and on the basis of their absolute velocity they should not be mistaken as being secondary to stenotic lesions. If there is doubt, the velocity proximal to the valve should be measured; if it is within 20 cm/s of the distal value there is not significant valve stenosis. In addition to increased flow, increased resistance to flow also produces a modest increase in velocity. For example, many patients with left ventricular outflow tract obstruction can have mitral velocities increased above two standard deviations from the mean. The importance of measuring velocity proximal to an obstruction, particularly in situations of high flow such as left to right shunts, must always be remembered if an accurate pressure gradient measurement is to be calculated using the Bernoulli equation.

Physiological tricuspid and pulmonary regurgitation

Tricuspid regurgitation

Tricuspid regurgitation may be detected using pulsed Doppler by sampling in the right atrium just posterior to the tricuspid valve leaflets. Because of the small size of the sample volume considerable manipulation of the transducer and the sample volume is required to detect even a qualitative signal. This is usually identified as turbulent flow of relatively high velocity directed away from the transducer. Signals may be obtained more easily using continuous wave Doppler, even without imaging, with the transducer placed as for recording normal tricuspid valve flow, i.e. just to the left of the lower sternal edge, and directed posteriorly. As yet there are no published normal values for tricuspid regurgitant velocity. The maximum velocity of this signal is related to the pressure difference between the right ventricle and atrium and thus if the maximum velocity can be measured it will be unusual for it to exceed 3 m/s (ventricular pressure less than 36 mmHg). Tricuspid regurgitation frequently may be found in completely normal subjects, but more commonly it occurs across a normal tricuspid valve in a heart which is diseased for other reasons, e.g. mitral or aortic valve disease.

Figure 3.8 demonstrates the typical qualitative waveform of tricuspid regurgitation which is relatively easy to obtain even in normal subjects. It is impossible to measure the peak velocity in this example. This so-called *physiological regurgitation* seems easier to obtain in adults with normal or diseased hearts than in children. In the paediatric population, tricuspid regurgitation may be detected across a normal valve particularly following ventricular surgery (i.e. when right bundle branch block is present), or in conditions with pulmonary hypertension and where the heart rate is slower. There are no firm rules as to which signals constitute pathological tricuspid regurgitation and at the moment there is probably no better way of distinguishing them than that pathological regurgitation gives an easily

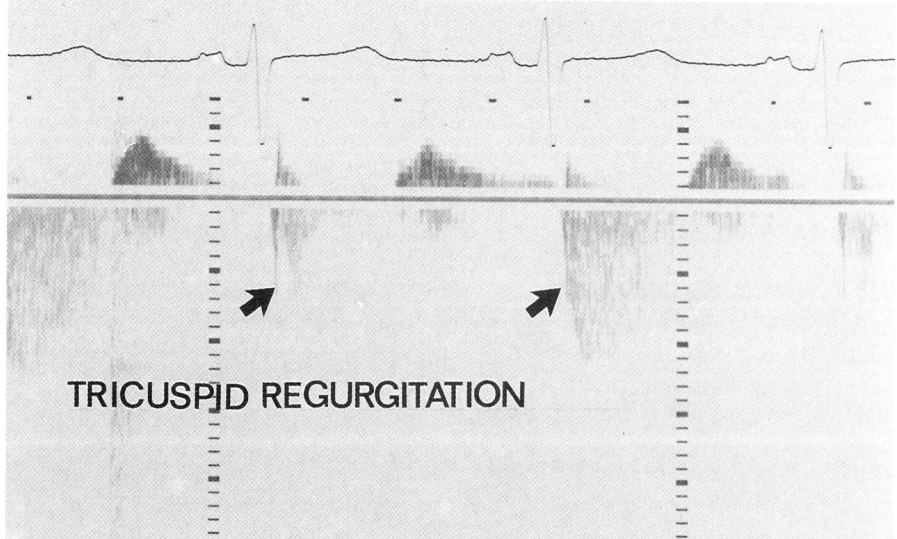

Figure 3.8 Typical tricuspid regurgitant waveform obtained from a normal subject. The time velocity waveform is incomplete and it is impossible to quantitate the peak velocity

detectable signal with a dense spectral display, though even this may be altered by gain settings. It is likely that if one has to search the right atrium for a long time to detect only a weak signal then the tricuspid regurgitation is likely to be trivial or physiological.

In those patients in whom the maximum velocity of tricuspid regurgitation can be measured, it is possible to make an assessment of right ventricular and thus pulmonary artery systolic pressure by applying the modified Bernoulli equation to the maximum velocity[11]; this gives the pressure drop from the right ventricle to atrium and if 5–10 mmHg is added to it for atrial pressure an estimate of the ventricular pressure is reached. This aspect of pulmonary artery pressure measurement is covered in more detail in Chapter 6.

Pulmonary regurgitation

It is common to find physiological pulmonary regurgitation, defined as a relatively weak low velocity signal detected proximal to a structurally normal pulmonary valve, either in a patient with completely normal cardiac anatomy or with pathology elsewhere in the heart but with a normal pulmonary valve. It is detected by imaging the pulmonary valve and main pulmonary artery in a standard short axis left parasternal view and placing the sample volume just proximal to the pulmonary valve. The maximum velocity of the Doppler signal obtained is usually in the region of 1.0–1.5 m/s and is directed towards the transducer. Interrogation of the pulmonary artery with continuous wave Doppler, even with a non-imaging transducer placed at the left parasternal edge and directed slightly cranially and posteriorly, will give a more easily detectable velocity waveform (*Figure 3.9*).

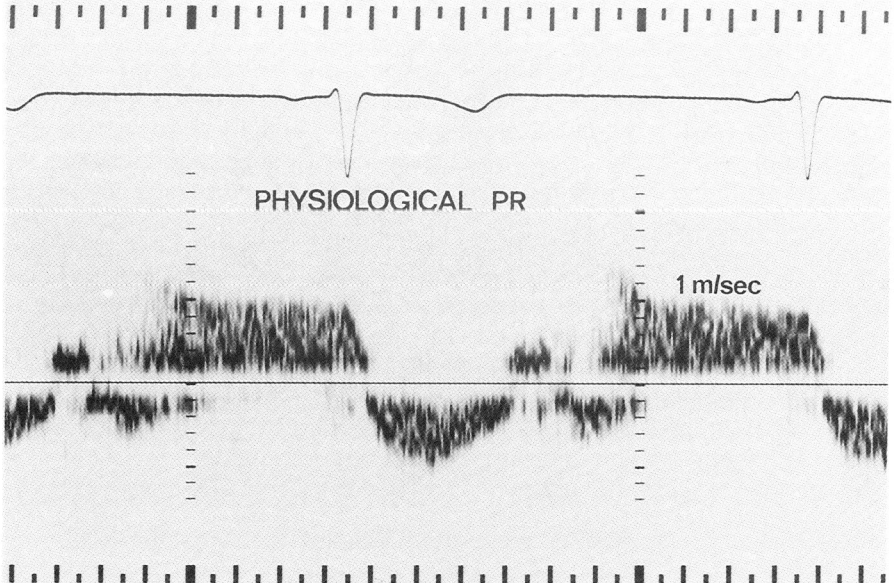

Figure 3.9 Pulmonary regurgitant waveform in a normal subject recorded with continuous wave Doppler from the left parasternal position. Low velocity diastolic flow directed towards the transducer. PR, pulmonary regurgitation

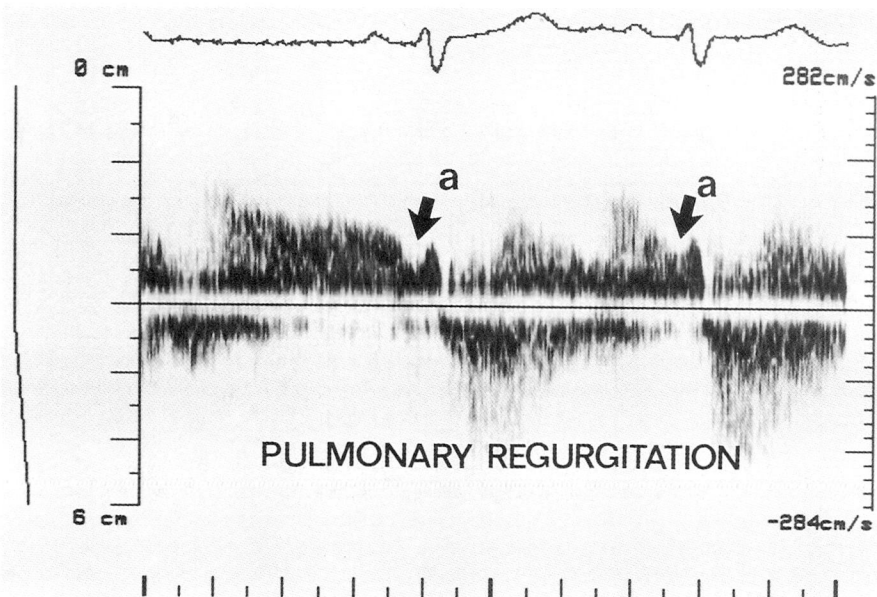

Figure 3.10 Pulmonary regurgitant time velocity waveform showing abruption of diastolic flow due to atrial contraction. There is a rapid decrease in the velocity of the regurgitant blood flow (arrowed a) immediately following the electrocardiographic P wave

With pandiastolic pulmonary regurgitation it is occasionally possible to identify a decrease in the waveform velocity corresponding to reduction of the regurgitant flow into the right ventricle as a result of atrial contraction (*Figure 3.10*). Once again the differentiation between physiological and pathological pulmonary regurgitation is on the basis of a normal valve on M-mode or two-dimensional study with a relatively weak regurgitant Doppler signal. Pulmonary regurgitation may be detected more easily in adults either with completely normal hearts or with pathology elsewhere in the heart. It is potentially possible to estimate the pulmonary artery diastolic pressure by calculating the diastolic gradient between the artery and ventricle by applying the modified Bernoulli equation to the maximum velocity of the regurgitant jet (*see* Chapter 7). As yet, however, there have been few if any correlative studies on the accuracy of this.

Conclusion

The ability to recognize the normal velocity patterns in the heart and great vessels is an important prerequisite for those performing a cardiac Doppler examination. Anyone learning the Doppler technique is encouraged to gain experience in sampling velocity patterns even in situations where flow patterns are expected to be normal. This will allow a confident approach in excluding variations of normality which may otherwise inadvertently be misconstrued as being abnormal. With care and experience the operator will avoid the mistakes that ambiguity and over-interpretation foster and the results obtained will be of great value and reassurance to both the operator and those clinicians referring patients for the study.

References

1. SEQUEIRA, R. F., LIGHT, L. H., CROSS, G. and RAFTERY, E. B. (1976) Transcutaneous aortovelography: a quantitative evaluation. *Br. Heart J.*, **38**, 443–450

2. MOWAT, D. H. R., HAITES, N. E. and RAWLES, J. M. (1983) Aortic blood velocity measurements in healthy adults using a simple ultrasound technique. *Cardiovas. Res.*, **17**, 75–80

3. HATLE, L. and ANGELSEN, B. (1985) *Doppler Ultrasound in Cardiology: Physical Principles and Clinical Applications*, 2nd edn, p. 93. Philadelphia: Lea and Febiger

4. GRENADIER, E., OLIVEIRA LIMA, C., ALLEN, H. D. *et al.* (1980) Normal intracardiac and great vessel Doppler flow velocities in infants and children. *J. Am. Coll. Cardiol.*, **4**, 343–350

5. WILSON, N., GOLDBERG, S. J., DICKINSON, D. F. and SCOTT, O. (1985) Normal intracardiac and great artery blood velocity measurements by pulsed Doppler echocardiography. *Br. Heart J.*, **53**, 451–458

6. HATLE, L. and ANGELSEN, B. *Doppler Ultrasound in Cardiology: Physical Principles and Clinical Applications*, 2nd edn, pp. 74–76. Philadelphia: Lea and Febiger

7. GIBBS, J. L., WILSON, N., WITSENBURG, M., WILLIAMS, G.J. and GOLDBERG, S. J. (1985) Diastolic forward blood flow in the pulmonary artery detected by Doppler echocardiography. *J. Am. Coll. Cardiol.*, **6**, 1322–1328

8. KOSTURAKIS, D., GOLDBERG, S. J., ALLEN, H. D. and LOEBER, C. (1984) Doppler echocardiographic prediction of pulmonary arterial hypertension in congenital heart disease. *Am. J. Cardiol.*, **53**, 1110–1115

9. KITABATAKE, A., INOUE, M., ASAO, M. *et al.* (1982) Transmitral blood flow reflecting diastolic behaviour of the left ventricle in health and disease. A study by pulsed Doppler. *Jpn. Circ. J.*, **46**, 92–102

10. GOLDBERG, S. J., WILSON, N. and DICKINSON, D. F. (1985) Increased blood velocities in the heart and great vessels of patients with congenital heart disease. An assessment of their significance in the absence of valvar stenosis. *Br. Heart J.*, **53**, 640–644

11. CURRIE, P. J., SEWARD, J. B., CHAN, K. L. *et al.* (1985) Continuous wave Doppler determination of right ventricular pressure: a simultaneous Doppler-catheterisation study in 127 patients. *J. Am. Coll. Cardiol.*, **6**, 750–756

4

Aortic valve disease

Donald J. Hagler

Aortic stenosis

The clinical assessment of the severity of aortic valve obstruction in both acquired rheumatic or calcific and congenital aortic valve stenosis has been notoriously unreliable. Symptoms related to the disease or the presence of a low pulse pressure indicate significant obstruction, but these appear late and in most patients the severity should be recognized earlier to allow appropriate surgical treatment. Until recently, the best non-invasive assessment was provided by the electrocardiogram (ECG); it was considered that obstruction of surgical significance did not occur without significant left ventricular hypertrophy and some would have considered strain the main indication for further investigation with a view to surgical treatment. However, severe aortic obstruction can occur with minimal changes in the ECG. Cardiac catheterization with haemodynamic measurement of aortic valve gradient has been the standard practice and the only reliable method for the assessment and follow-up of such patients. However, it is not always possible to cross the aortic valve at catheterization and direct left ventricular or trans-septal puncture to measure the left ventricular pressure is not without hazard. Furthermore, in order to decide on appropriate therapy several cardiac catheterization procedures may be necessary over a period to follow the severity of stenosis, particularly in children and adolescents during rapid growth phases. Clearly, an accurate non-invasive means of predicting the severity of aortic valve stenosis would considerably improve and simplify assessment and long-term follow-up.

Standard M-mode and two-dimensional echocardiographic measurements of chamber size and wall dimensions do provide valuable and useful information to assess the severity of left ventricular enlargement and hypertrophy and these should form the basis of the echocardiographic study in aortic stenosis. In addition, they can provide valuable structural information by identifying thickening and calcification of the aortic cusps, aortic valve prolapse and the presence of a bicuspid aortic valve. There can be considerable difficulty in assessing the degree of stenosis from the appearance of the valve particularly where calcification is present and indeed the presence of calcification does not necessarily imply obstruction. Therefore the effect of the obstruction on the left ventricle is of more importance in assessing the severity of stenosis.

Concentric left ventricular hypertrophy in the presence of an abnormal aortic valve is highly suggestive of significant stenosis but this may be invalid in hypertensive patients or where alternative reasons for ventricular hypertrophy exist. In children and adolescents, an estimation of left ventricular systolic pressure (LVP) can be obtained from measurement of the end systolic left ventricular wall thickness (LVWT) and internal dimension (LVID) from the formula:

$$LVP = LVWT/LVID \times 245[1]$$

Although echocardiography may reveal cases of significant aortic stenosis not suspected on other grounds, it mainly separates those with severe as opposed to minimal obstruction and is of limited value in those of intermediate severity where ECG and clinical examination are inconclusive.

With aortic regurgitation, echocardiography can suggest its presence from mitral valve flutter or premature closure and give some idea of its severity by assessing left ventricular dimensions and function. However, difficulties arise in patients with multivalve disease, heart failure, or wall motion abnormalities following myocardial infarction. Indeed, although many patients with valvar heart disease can safely undergo valve replacement without prior cardiac catheterization[2] it seems that aortic stenosis, particularly calcific aortic stenosis, is the one lesion where the need for surgery cannot be safely predicted on the basis of a complete non-invasive assessment with history, clinical examination, ECG, chest X-ray and echocardiography[3].

Recently, the development and application of pulsed and continuous wave Doppler ultrasound have demonstrated the value of Doppler echocardiography for non-invasive assessment of aortic valve disease[4] and, for aortic stenosis, these other techniques are relatively insensitive by comparison and have, to an extent, been superseded.

Measurement of gradient

Technique

The basic principle in determining the severity of aortic stenosis is that the maximum flow velocity through the narrowed area is measured with Doppler and the Bernoulli equation used to calculate the pressure drop across it (*Figure 4.1*). Doppler techniques and instrumentation are extremely varied and each has a different role in the assessment of aortic valve disease. For precise placement of the sample volume pulsed Doppler studies are required and, for practical purposes, are best combined with duplex imaging capabilities. The high velocities which occur with significant aortic stenosis preclude its use in measuring the gradient exactly, but some instruments allowing high pulsed repetition rates have improved the results of such pulsed Doppler studies. Although the site of obstruction is usually apparent on echocardiography, pulsed Doppler interrogation of the left ventricular outflow tract is worthwhile to rule out subaortic obstruction and, in addition, is essential for calculating aortic valve area and may be helpful in recognizing the presence of aortic regurgitation.

Pulsed Doppler interrogation of the subaortic velocity is best performed from the cardiac apex to allow parallel orientation of the ultrasonic beam to aortic flow. The sample volume is moved progressively from the body of the left ventricle to the

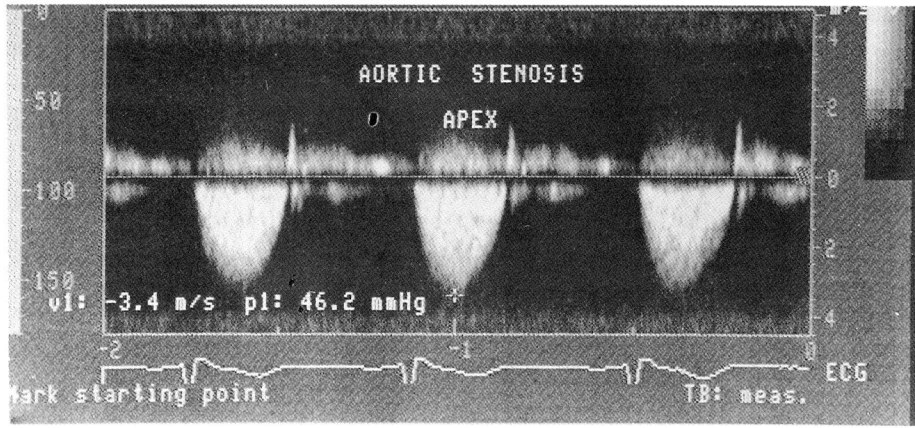

(a)

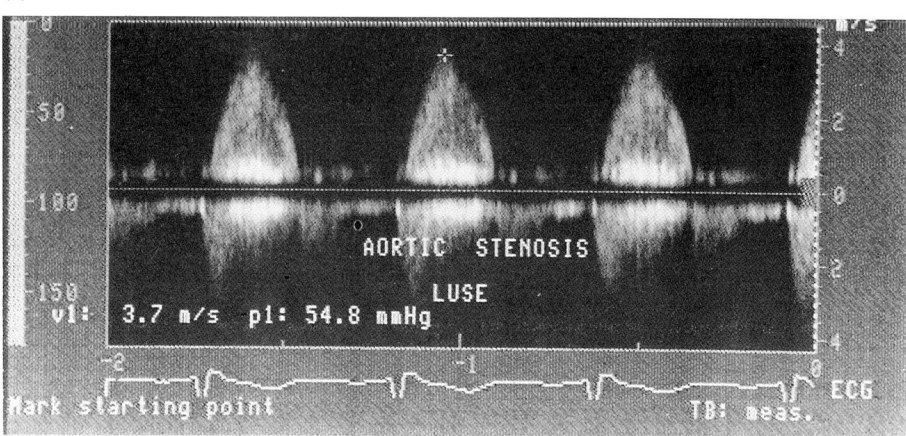

(b)

Figure 4.1 Doppler recordings made from (*a*) the apex and (*b*) the left upper parasternal edge (LUSE) in a 10-year-old boy with aortic stenosis. The flow signal is systolic with maximum velocity in mid-systole. The maximum velocity (3.7 m/s corresponding to a maximum instantaneous gradient of 55 mmHg) is obtained from the left parasternal edge, indicating optimal alignment with the jet from this site

outflow area and through the aortic valve to the ascending aorta. Where duplex imaging is not available, it is possible, with practice, to determine the position of the sample volume from the flow signal and valve clicks; in the subvalve area the closing valve movement is recorded, and as the sample volume is moved to the valve orifice the opening also becomes apparent. Most often continuous wave rather than high pulse repetition Doppler measurement is necessary to provide optimal signals of the high velocities (i.e. greater than 4 m/s) found with significant aortic stenosis or regurgitation.

Since precise localization of the direction of the jet is not apparent from the two-dimensional image the use of a duplex system is of limited value in determining the correct alignment of the beam and may even be misleading. Thus, even if the continuous wave transducer is interfaced to an imaging system, the preferred methodology is to use all possible precordial sampling sites to obtain the highest velocity possible and minimize the risk of false low recordings with consequent underestimation of gradient. It is recommended that maximum flow velocity is measured from apical, subcostal, left parasternal, right parasternal (often best with the patient in the right lateral decubitus position), right supraclavicular, and suprasternal positions. In children, good signals can usually be obtained from all these sites but, in older patients, the choice may be more limited and the apex may be the only one from which a satisfactory recording can be obtained. The variability in Doppler signals recorded from different sites is shown in *Figure 4.1*. Angulation of the Doppler beam is often easier with a small non-imaging transducer and in each position it should be redirected until the operator detects the highest pitched audible velocity signal to assist in obtaining the highest spectral display and allow more precise detection of the maximum velocity for gradient prediction. When available, colour flow imaging may allow localization of the jets and placement of the Doppler beam, but multiple sampling sites are again advised.

When this methodology is followed, optimal signals are presumed to have been obtained with the beam almost parallel to the direction of maximal blood flow velocity across the stenosis and the highest velocity obtained from any site is then used to calculate the pressure gradient. Therefore no correction is used to compensate for any presumed angle between the ultrasound beam and the direction of the maximal systolic jet. The Doppler determined estimate of systolic pressure gradient across the aortic valve is then calculated from the modified Bernoulli equation as:

$$\text{gradient} = 4V^2$$

where gradient equals the maximum instantaneous pressure gradient in mmHg and V^2 equals the maximum Doppler velocity (in m/s) squared.

Problems in application

The ability of continuous wave Doppler reliably and accurately to predict the transvalvar gradient in aortic stenosis is well proven. Although most reported studies have suggested a reasonable correlation between the outpatient Doppler predicted gradient and that subsequently measured by catheter withdrawal, the two measurements are not strictly comparable. An outpatient result cannot simply be used to replace the standard measurement by catheter withdrawal but must be interpreted in the light of the factors which may modify it. The three main factors are variation in gradient with time, unreliability of withdrawal as opposed to dual catheter measurements, and difference between peak-to-peak and instantaneous gradients.

Considerable variability in haemodynamic measurements occurs with changes in the patient's state of activity and sedation; a gradient obtained from someone who is apprehensive at an outpatient visit is likely to be higher than that at catheterization, particularly if this is performed under general anaesthesia. A detailed and important study of 100 adult patients[5] has reinforced the need for simultaneous measurements for accurate comparative studies, confirming the variability in gradients with time which is clearly apparent on Doppler studies. Furthermore, this study also highlighted the other problems in comparing the two techniques. It is clear that the gradient measured on withdrawal does not accurately compare with that measured more precisely by the use of a dual catheter system

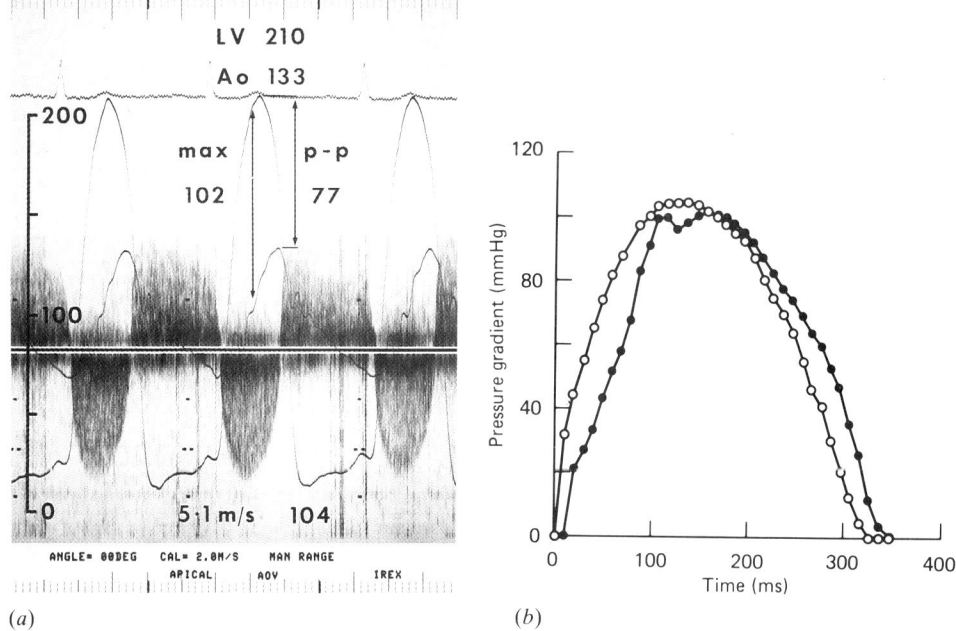

Figure 4.2 (*a*) Simultaneous recording of aortic valve gradient and continuous wave Doppler velocity (obtained from the apex) across the left ventricular outflow tract obtained during cardiac catheterization. The aortic valve gradient is instantaneously recorded with a dual catheter technique allowing identification of maximum instantaneous, peak, and mean pressure gradients. The Doppler velocity of 5.1 m/s gives a gradient of 104 mmHg which compares more favourably with the measured instantaneous (102 mmHg) than the peak-to-peak. Note also the diastolic flow towards the transducer due to aortic regurgitation. (*b*) Computer display of Doppler (open dots) and catheter (closed dots) derived pressure gradients. The gradient is displayed in 10 ms time increments. Note the slight phase shift due to delayed pressure transmission through the fluid-filled catheter system. Maximum instantaneous gradients correspond closely. The Doppler mean gradient can be calculated from this display of Doppler gradient from the area under the curve and the duration of the flow signal

with one proximal and the other distal to the obstructive lesion in order to measure exactly the pressure difference across the valve and demonstrate changes in it with time. Perhaps more importantly, this technique has demonstrated that, although continuous wave Doppler does accurately predict transvalvar aortic gradient, this represents the maximal instantaneous rather than the peak-to-peak gradient usually measured and clinically utilized. However, it did show that continuous wave Doppler measurement of the mean aortic valve gradient correlated well with that measured by cardiac catheterization.

This is a very important concept in understanding and interpreting Doppler measured gradients and is nicely demonstrated in *Figure 4.2a*. By using the dual catheter technique recordings of left ventricular and aortic pressure tracings were recorded simultaneously on the same strip as the continuous wave Doppler spectral velocities. Instantaneous Doppler and catheter pressure gradients were then calculated at 10 ms intervals and plotted against each other (*Figure 4.2b*). Doppler determined mean gradients were derived from the instantaneous Doppler determined gradients during systole. The maximum gradient measured by catheter

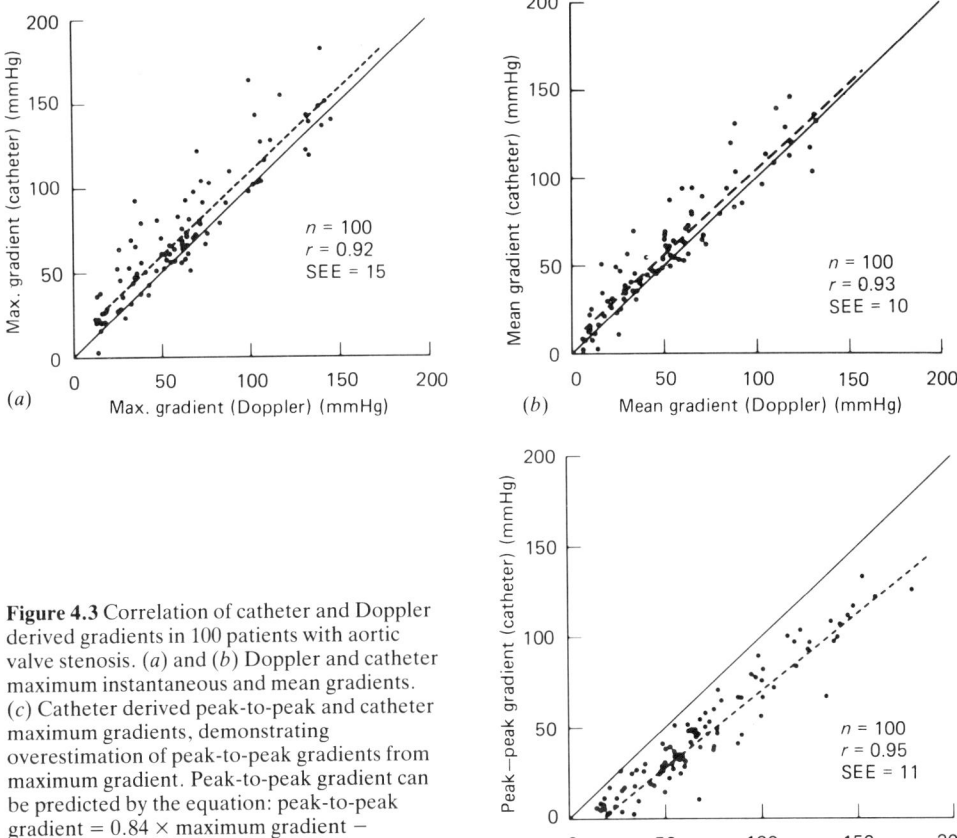

Figure 4.3 Correlation of catheter and Doppler derived gradients in 100 patients with aortic valve stenosis. (*a*) and (*b*) Doppler and catheter maximum instantaneous and mean gradients. (*c*) Catheter derived peak-to-peak and catheter maximum gradients, demonstrating overestimation of peak-to-peak gradients from maximum gradient. Peak-to-peak gradient can be predicted by the equation: peak-to-peak gradient = 0.84 × maximum gradient − 13.7 mmHg. (From Currie, *et al*.[5] by permission of the American Heart Association)

was the maximum instantaneous gradient between the left ventricle and ascending aorta and the peak-to-peak systolic gradient was the difference between the peak systolic pressures in the left ventricle and ascending aorta. Thus, peak-to-peak pressure gradients do not represent the maximum instantaneous gradients derived from the maximum Doppler velocity. Using this method, catheter derived pressure gradients can be compared to Doppler derived instantaneous gradients on a beat-to-beat basis.

In the study by Currie *et al*.[5] of 100 patients with aortic valve stenosis, there was a good correlation between both the maximum (*Figure 4.3a*) and mean (*Figure 4.3b*) catheter and Doppler gradients. The peak-to-peak gradient measured by catheter was significantly lower than the maximum catheter gradient or the maximum Doppler determined gradient. Although the correlation between the maximum Doppler gradient and peak-to-peak catheter gradient was satisfactory, with an *r* value of 0.91 and a standard error of the estimate of 14 mmHg, the measured maximum instantaneous catheter gradient was always higher than the peak-to-peak over a wide range of severity of aortic stenosis. Thus gradient derived from the maximum velocity better corresponds to the maximum instantaneous gradient which is greater than the peak-to-peak difference over a wide range of

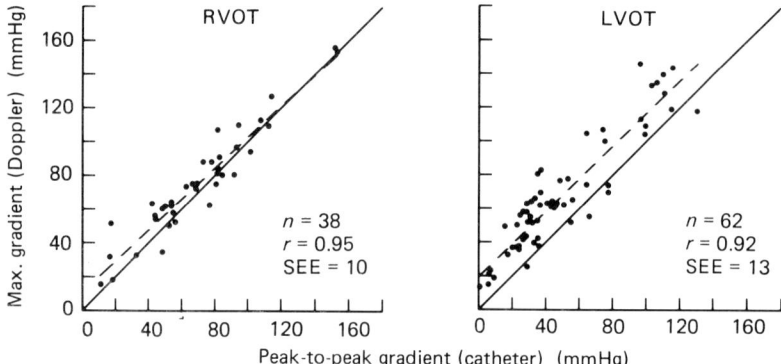

Figure 4.4 Correlation of catheter and Doppler derived maximum instantaneous gradients in 100 children with right (RVOT) or left ventricular outflow tract obstruction (LVOT). Note that while the Doppler velocity accurately predicts the peak-to-peak right ventricular outflow gradients, the peak-to-peak left ventricular outflow gradients are significantly overestimated. SEE standard error of the estimate. (From Currie *et al*.[6] by permission of the American College of Cardiology)

severity of aortic stenosis, but is greatest in the mild to moderate lesions, i.e. Doppler tends to overestimate peak-to-peak gradient. Similar findings occur in children[6], but it is noteworthy that although left ventricular outflow tract peak-to-peak gradients are overestimated, as is discussed in Chapter 7, continuous wave Doppler accurately predicts the measured peak-to-peak right ventricular outflow tract gradients (*Figure 4.4*).

Thus Doppler estimated gradient will be somewhat higher than the peak-to-peak at catheterization (*see Figure 4.3c*); in the future it is likely that the Doppler maximum or mean gradient will be accepted on its own merit but, in the meantime, if it is felt appropriate to attempt to translate this to a peak-to-peak gradient a variety of techniques have been suggested. The regression equation derived from Currie's study can be employed:

Peak-to-peak gradient = 0.84 × maximum gradient − 13.7 mmHg (*Figure 4.3c*)

A gradient derived from the average of the peak gradient and the systolic gradient at two-thirds of the ventricular ejection time can also be employed[7].

Two separate studies of an experimental dog model of aortic stenosis also documented the excellent correlation between maximum Doppler and maximum instantaneous pressure gradients[8, 9], with Doppler systematically overestimating the peak-to-peak pressure gradient. The beat-to-beat relationship of these gradients in an open chest dog preparation where supravalvar aortic stenosis was created is clearly shown in *Figure 4.5*. The study by Smith *et al*.[9] also suggested that measurement of the Doppler gradient at mid-systole resulted in more accurate correlation with peak-to-peak catheterization gradient and this might eliminate the problem of overestimation (*Figure 4.6*).

The shape of the Doppler velocity recording may also be valuable in assessing the severity of aortic obstruction. In normal aortic flow or in mild aortic obstruction the peak velocity occurs early in systole, whereas in severe obstruction this peak velocity occurs later, in mid-systole. Although this is somewhat subjective, it may be important with critical aortic stenosis and severe left ventricular dysfunction where the aortic valve gradient may be relatively low, or when difficulty is encountered in obtaining good quality spectral records.

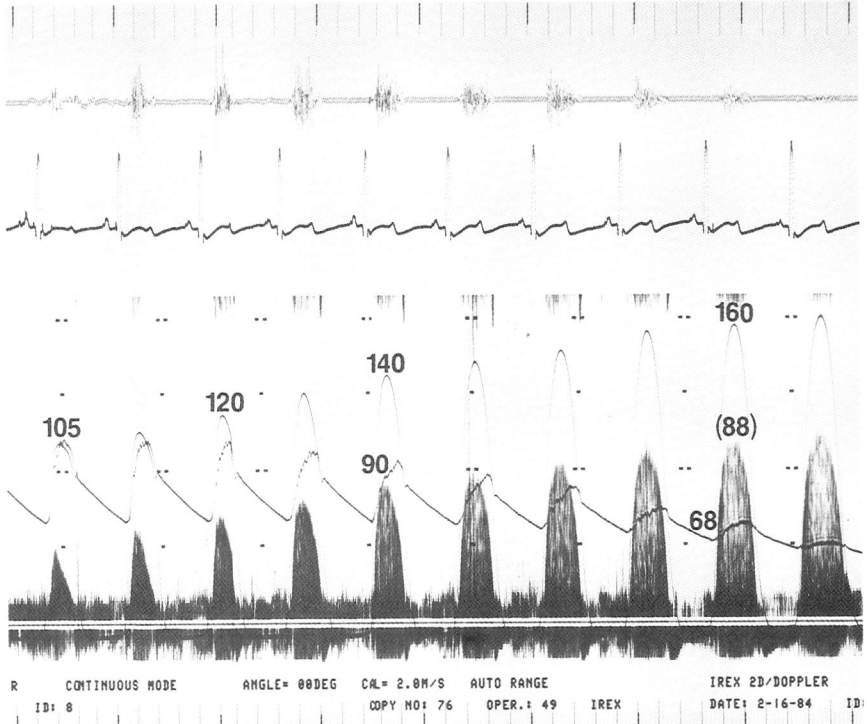

Figure 4.5 Record obtained at a paper speed of 25 mm/s during progressive tightening of the ascending aortic snare. Vertical dots are the Doppler velocity calibration in 2 m/s intervals. Peak left ventricular (LV) systolic pressures are recorded above the LV traces. Simultaneous aortic pressures are recorded next to the aortic traces. The maximal Doppler derived gradient for the next to last cycle is recorded in parentheses next to the aortic pressure trace. Note the concurrent increase in both the catheter gradient and the Doppler velocity, on a beat-to-beat basis. At the start of the recording, peak LV systolic pressure is 105 mmHg with a minimal gradient. At this point, the peak Doppler velocity is 1.7 m/s, which yields a maximal instantaneous gradient of 11 mmHg. The snare is then tightened. Near the end of the recording, the maximal instantaneous catheter gradient is 92 mmHg with a peak LV systolic pressure of 160 mmHg. The maximal Doppler velocity at this time is 4.7 m/s. This yields a maximal gradient of 88 mmHg. (From Callahan *et al.*[8] by permission of the *American Journal of Cardiology*)

Aortic valve area

The pressure gradient is most often used to assess the severity of aortic stenosis but its level varies with flow across it and may be misleading where this is abnormal. Thus in critical aortic stensois with left ventricular dysfunction and poor cardiac output the gradient may be relatively low, while with moderate stenosis and aortic regurgitation the increased forward flow can produce an apparently significant gradient. Calculation of valve area then becomes of importance and hopefully may remove some of the concerns related to gradient calculation, particularly overestimation in the presence of significant aortic regurgitation. Two techniques have been described for the estimation of aortic valve area with Doppler, but only limited clinical experience is currently available and, as yet, their value is uncertain.

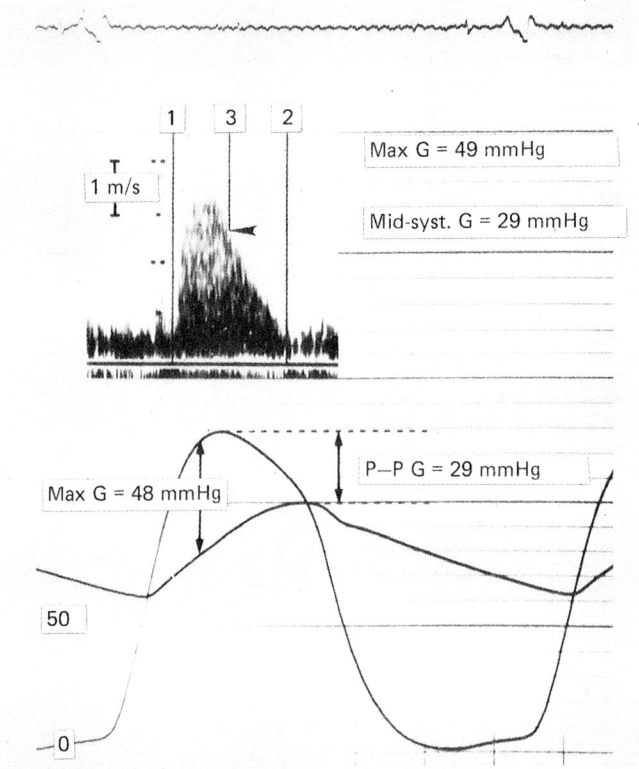

Figure 4.6 Simultaneous recorded catheter and Doppler velocity in an open chest dog with a surgically placed supravalvar aortic band, demonstrating correlation of maximum instantaneous catheter and Doppler derived gradients (G). In addition, the peak-to-peak gradient is predicted from the Doppler velocity at mid-systole. (From Smith *et al.*[9] by permission of the American College of Cardiology)

It is possible to calculate the aortic valve area with Doppler by applying it to the classical Gorlin equation[10, 11]:

$$\text{Aortic valve area (area AV)} = \frac{\text{cardiac output}}{44.5 \times \text{SEP} \times \sqrt{\text{MTG}}}$$

Cardiac output (CO) is derived in the left ventricular outflow tract from measurement of the systolic velocity integral by pulsed Doppler and the cross-sectional area from two-dimensional echocardiography (*Figure 4.7*)[12] as described in Chapter 10. The systolic ejection period (SEP) is derived by multiplying the heart rate by the aortic ejection time, defined non-invasively as the time interval between the aortic valve opening and closure signals on the continuous wave aortic Doppler tracing. Mean transaortic pressure gradient (MTG) is determined from the modified Bernoulli equation. A further, slightly more complicated, modification of this can be employed to obviate the need for area measurement[10].

The other method for the determination of valve area employs the so-called continuity equation[12, 13], the fact that the stroke volume in the outflow tract (LVOT) equals that through the aortic orifice (AV). Area is measured by echocardiography and the systolic velocity integral (SVI) from Doppler by

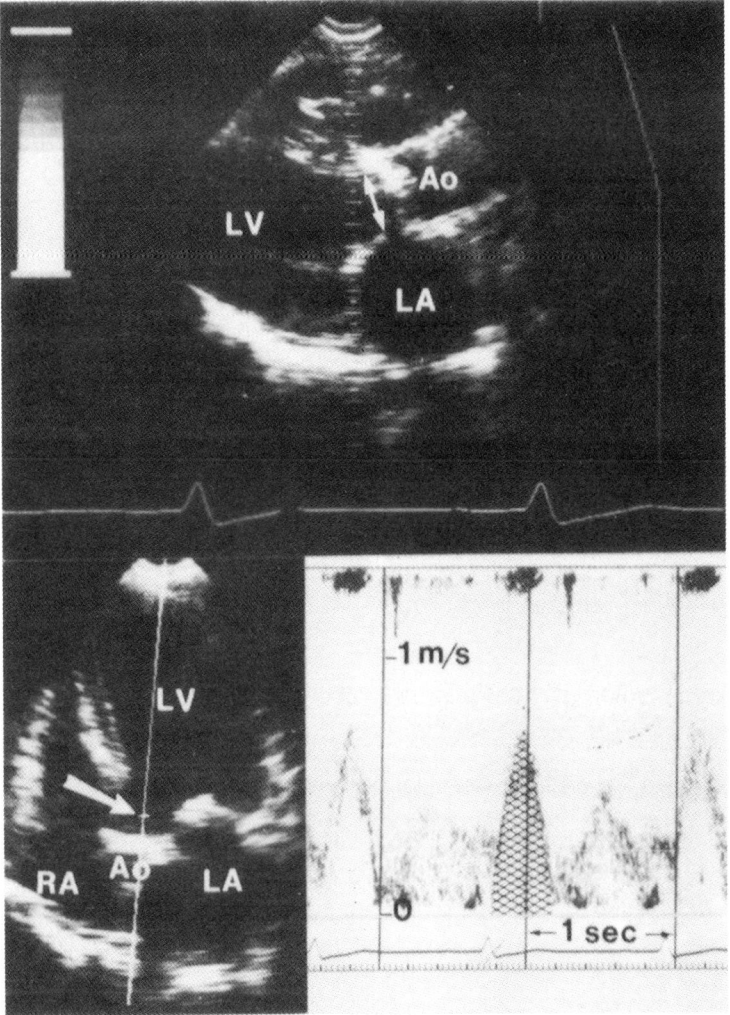

Figure 4.7 Technique for measuring cardiac output. The left ventricular outflow tract diameter is measured from a long axis view (arrows) and the systolic velocity integral is obtained from the area enclosed by the hatch marks with the sample volume just proximal to the aortic valve. LV, left ventricle; LA, left atrium; Ao, aorta. (From Otto *et al.*[12] by permission of the American College of Cardiology

determination of the area enclosed by the Doppler spectral display envelope (*Figure 4.7*).

Thus: area LVOT $\times$ SVI LVOT = area AV $\times$ SVI AV

and: area AV $=\dfrac{\text{area LVOT} \times \text{SVI LVOT}}{\text{SVI AV}}$

Although a good correlation ($r = 0.88$) has been found between the aortic valve area determined by Doppler and catheter methods, there is considerable variation between them, and its routine use in clinical practice is as yet unproved.

Aortic regurgitation

With pulsed Doppler aortic regurgitation can best be recognized in the immediate subvalve area as retrograde flow through the aortic valve or, when of moderate or severe degree, also as diastolic flow reversal in the proximal aorta. Regurgitant diastolic flow in the left ventricular outflow tract is more easily obtained with continuous wave Doppler which, in any case, is usually required to demonstrate clearly the high velocities and full spectral signal; maximum flow velocity occurs early with subsequent reduction throughout diastole as aortic and ventricular pressures become more equal (*Figures 4.2* and *4.8*). The position and angulation from which forward flow is best obtained is not necessarily the optimal one for finding aortic regurgitation and again multiple positions similar to those used for aortic stenosis should be explored before the presence of aortic regurgitation can be excluded.

The quantitation of aortic regurgitation using the present non-invasive techniques is difficult and even on angiocardiography can only be labelled mild, moderate or severe. Doppler is a sensitive way of detecting aortic regurgitation, and can also be applied in the assessment of its severity. A simple assessment of gross degrees (mild, moderate and severe) of aortic valve insufficiency is obtained by mapping the extension of the regurgitant jet into the ventricle with pulsed Doppler. This is best performed from an apical position with an imaging transducer demonstrating the body and outflow tract of the left ventricle. The sample volume is progressively moved back from the valve area into the body of the ventricle to determine the distance to which the regurgitant jet extends. When the distance to the valve is large or high pulse repetition frequency Doppler is used care should be exercised to ensure that range ambiguity inherent in the system does not give a false impression of the extent of regurgitation. This basic technique has been simplified more recently by the use of two-dimensional Doppler colour flow mapping to assess the extent of aortic regurgitation from the size and length of the regurgitant jet into the left ventricular cavity (*see Plate 1*). By using multiple parasternal long and short axis views as well as that of the apical long axis, an estimate of the regurgitation (mild, moderate and severe) has corresponded to angiographic assessment of the regurgitant flow.

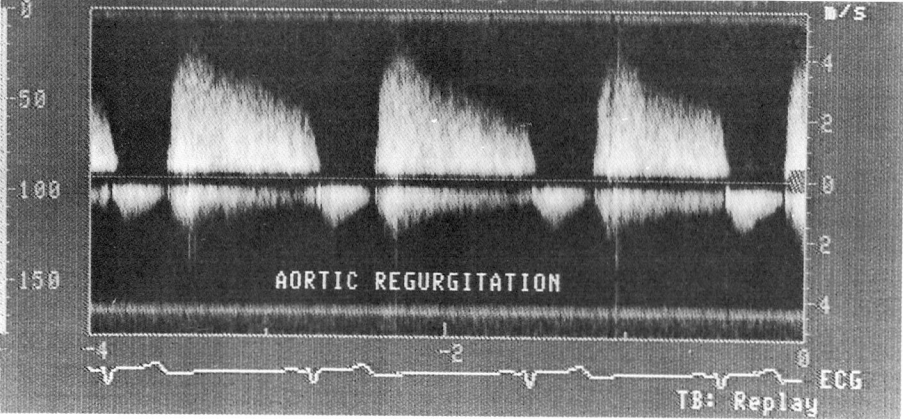

Figure 4.8 Recording from an apical position from a patient with aortic regurgitation. The signal has maximum velocity early and shows a progressive fall in the diastolic velocity indicating mild to moderate regurgitation

Continuous wave Doppler can give an idea of the severity from the flow pattern since this reflects the pressure difference across the aortic valve throughout diastole; with mild regurgitation the pressure difference changes little and the velocity remains almost the same while in severe regurgitation the maximal velocity of aortic valve insufficiency decreases rapidly because the pressure difference between the aorta and the left ventricle diminishes[4]. However, this information is similar to that obtained from measurement of pulse pressure. The intensity of the continuous wave Doppler signal tends to increase with the amount of regurgitation and can give a clue to its degree; since the intensity recorded will vary with gain settings this is a somewhat subjective technique.

If a pulsed sample volume is positioned in the aortic arch the signal will demonstrate retrograde diastolic flow as the blood runs back into the ventricle. This is not usually apparent with mild regurgitation, but should increase as the regurgitation increases. Quantitation of both forward and backward flow is difficult since the pulsatile nature of the aorta at this position makes area measurement difficult. Nevertheless, attempts to correlate the ratio of forward and reverse flow in the upper descending aorta have shown that it is possible[14]. Alternatively, a regurgitant fraction can be calculated by comparing right and left ventricular stroke volume[15]. These are measured non-invasively by echocardiographic and Doppler interrogation of their outflow tracts. Where there is no shunt the stroke volume (SV) through the aorta equals that through the pulmonary artery and for each site:

$$SV = \pi \times radius^2 \times SVI \text{ (systolic velocity integral).}$$

$$\text{The regurgitant fraction} = \frac{Lt\ SV - Rt\ SV}{Lt\ SV} \times 100$$

This method seems fairly reliable when isolated aortic regurgitation is studied and when compared to catheterization methods using ventriculography and thermo-dilution a correlation coefficient of 0.96 was obtained[15].

Clinical application

It has been suggested that the non-invasive assessment of valve disease can obviate the need for cardiac catheterization in many cases[2]. However, patients with aortic stenosis are often the most difficult to assess by non-invasive means, and cardiac catheterization is almost always required. It is important to emphasize that, especially in adult patients with aortic stenosis, difficulty may be encountered in obtaining satisfactory Doppler recordings and considerable experience and patience is required to identify the high velocity jet at a low intercept angle, and even more so to exclude the presence of a higher velocity jet. To this end a small non-imaging continuous wave transducer is easier to manipulate and often more sensitive than one incorporated in a duplex scanner. In any individual patient it is important to interrogate multiple praecordial positions some of which are not recognized for imaging, and there will therefore be a substantial learning curve even for those experienced in echocardiography.

Although measurement of aortic valve orifice area is a more exact means of assessment of the severity of aortic stenosis, for practical purposes the gradient is measured and its significance determined in the light of other clinical or investigative findings. The correlation found between the Doppler derived gradient and that obtained at catheterization indicates that Doppler ultrasound can provide an accurate assessment of the gradient across an aortic obstruction. For those with limited experience of Doppler it must be emphasized that the relationship of Doppler derived gradients with invasive pressure measurements may be appreciably affected by the relative time of the studies and the fact that, up till now, at catheterization peak-to-peak systolic gradients have conventionally been measured rather than the maximum instantaneous or mean gradient as measured by the Doppler technique. An outpatient value is likely to be higher than a measured one because of the effect of sedation and the fact that Doppler measures instantaneous not peak-to-peak gradient. Doppler ultrasound should not significantly overestimate the maximum instantaneous pressure gradient in patients with aortic stenosis, particularly if account is taken of the velocity proximal to the obstruction, so that it should be possible to comment that the actual instantaneous pressure gradient is at least as high as that derived from Doppler examination.

The application of the Doppler derived mean aortic valve gradients may provide additional information for clinical assessment of severity of stenosis. Thus a false high prediction of peak-to-peak aortic valve gradient from the Doppler maximum instantaneous gradient may be obviated by recognition of an associated low mean gradient. Nevertheless, it can be argued that by attempting to measure a very small high velocity jet at an unknown angle, the possibility of obtaining false low pressure gradients by the Doppler technique must exist. It will be related not only to the suitability of the patient for ultrasound study, but also to the expertise of the investigator in obtaining signals from a number of different sites. Therefore extreme care should be taken in interpreting the result of a Doppler examination that suggests a less than significant obstruction where this is at variance with either the clincial or routine non-invasive examinations. Where there is any doubt other factors should be taken into consideration in deciding the appropriate course of action. The measurement of aortic valve area and estimation of peak-to-peak pressure with Doppler may be of value in doubtful cases, but as yet more experience is required in their practical application.

More important than the accurate correlation of valve gradients with catheterization data is the ability of the Doppler technique to help determine the appropriate clinical management of the patient with aortic stenosis when integrated as part of a complete non-invasive assessment. No patient with a surgically significant lesion should be missed by complete non-invasive assessment including Doppler examination, and in none should there be an appreciable overestimation of the severity of obstruction providing the problems in the technique are considered[16]. Where doubt exists as to the severity of a lesion by other non-invasive techniques alone, Doppler examination should be able correctly to clarify the degree of obstruction. The Doppler examination can be of particular value in identifying patients with surgically significant lesions which would otherwise have been missed by routine clinical and non-invasive assessment.

In a number of patients with no demonstrable valve gradient at catheterization, Doppler ultrasound can suggest the presence of a small, though clearly non-significant, transvalvar gradient. It is likely that this results from failure of the modified Bernoulli formula to take into account the flow velocity proximal to the valve and this may occur particularly in patients with aortic regurgitation where flow through the aortic valve is increased. This would cause a higher peak velocity to be present and therefore suggest a degree of obstruction from the modified Bernoulli equation. Alternatively, a small instantaneous gradient may be present,

Plate 1 Parasternal long (LAx) and short (SAx) axis and apical long axis colour flow mapping views demonstrating moderate aortic valve insufficiency. Aliasing occurs in the jet causing a mosaic of colours. LV, left ventricle; LA, left atrium; AR, aortic root

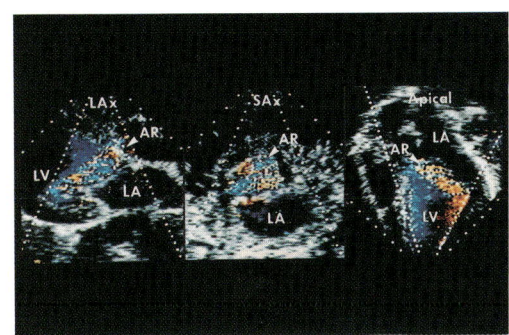

Plate 2 Apical long axis view in systole (left) and diastole (right) of a normal subject. During systole flow is away from the transducer and encoded in blue. Note the increasing brightness indicating an increasing velocity in the left ventricular outflow tract until the colour changes into yellow/red as a result of the aliasing phenomenon when the velocity exceeds the Nyquist limit. During diastole left ventricular inflow is towards the transducer and encoded in red. Note the turbulence at the tip of the anterior mitral valve leaflet, which is a normal phenomenon

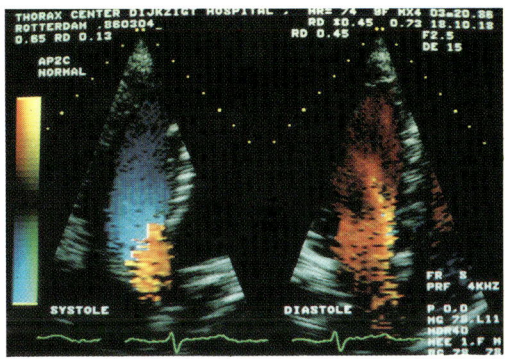

Plate 3 Colour-coded and continuous wave Doppler study in a patient with mitral stenosis and atrial fibrillation. The stenotic jet is visualized and bends off towards the inferolateral wall of the left ventricle. Central aliasing of the high velocities in the middle of the stenotic jet, which are encoded in blue, creates a 'flame-shaped' appearance of the jet. Continuous wave Doppler sampling is performed along a sound beam indicated on the flow map and the spectral velocity output is shown to the left. The angle between the jet flow and sound beam can be adjusted on the flow map allowing an accurate calculation of blood velocity. As an example, the velocity has been measured in early diastole (indicated by the cursor on the spectral velocity output in blue) and automatically calculated by machine software. The peak velocity (VP) in this beat is 2.09 m/s representing a pressure difference (PG) of 24 mm at that particular moment in diastole. It should be realized that a change in transducer position and a better jet direction/sound beam alignment is preferable to angle correction for accurate velocity measurement but this is not always possible in the clinical situation

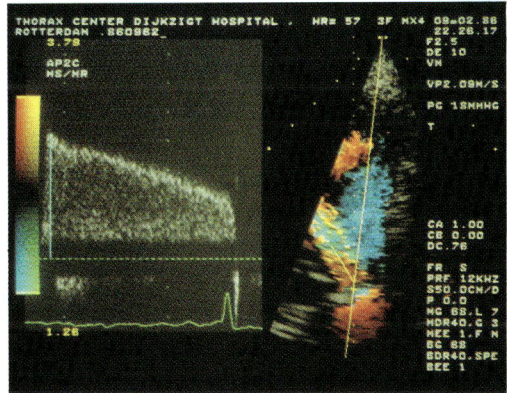

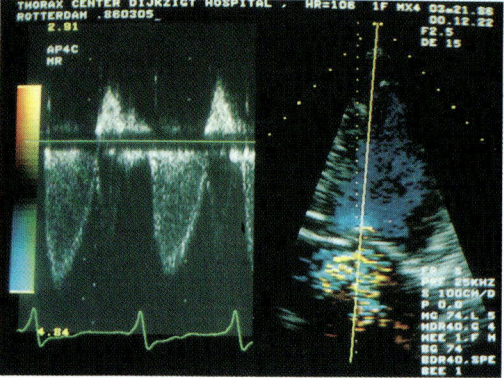

Plate 4 Colour and continuous wave Doppler study of mitral regurgitation. Two turbulent jets are posterior to the mitral valve arising from the same central defect (right). The continuous wave Doppler trace (left) shows a waveform consistent with severe mitral regurgitation where the pressure differences rapidly decrease during systole, resulting in a rapidly decreasing blood flow velocity

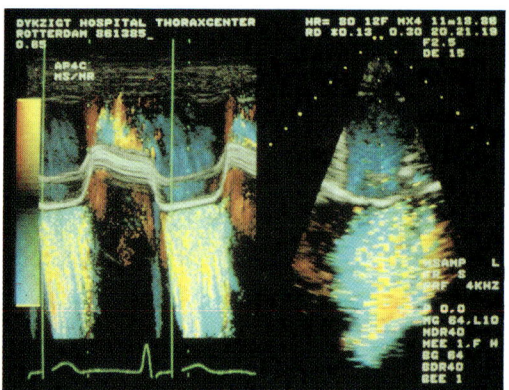

Plate 5 A systolic apical four chamber view of a patient with mitral valve disease. Note the wide area and extent of turbulent flow in the left atrium confirming severe mitral regurgitation. A single Doppler line is selected and indicated on the flow map. The blood flow velocity and its dispersion at each point along this interrogating Doppler beam axis is displayed in colour and superimposed on the M-mode mitral valve echocardiogram (left) which demonstrates the typical pattern of mitral stenosis. The regurgitant jet is displayed posterior to the mitral valve and the exact timing of the regurgitant flow can be analysed

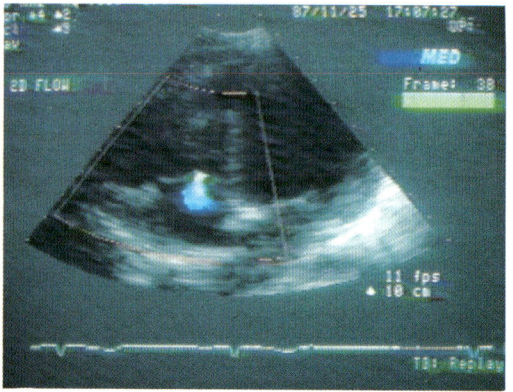

Plate 6 Colour Doppler flow image from a subject with a normal heart demonstrating physiological tricuspid regurgitation. The regurgitant jet originates at the point of apposition of the cusps and extends for only a short distance into the right atrium

Plate 7 Colour flow study demonstrating the tricuspid regurgitation jet and the distance it extends into the right atrium. The spectral display is that of severe regurgitation with rapid fall in the velocities

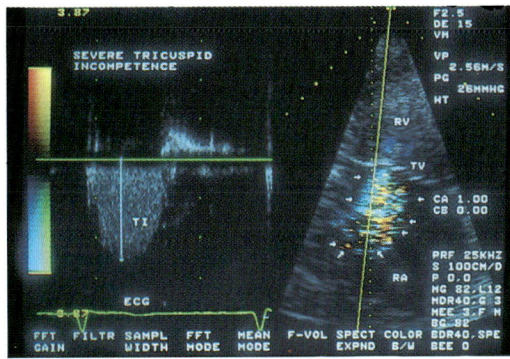

Plate 8 Colour flow image demonstrating the clear signal from retrograde flow of blood from the right atrium into the inferior vena cava (IVC) and hepatic veins

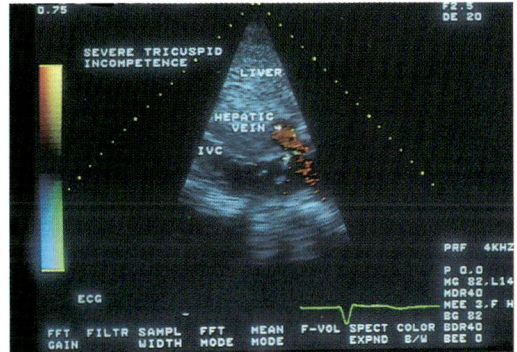

Plate 9 Parasternal short axis view at the level of the main pulmonary artery (MPA) in diastole showing a narrow stream of red diastolic regurgitant flow across the pulmonary valve leaflets. RVOT, right ventricular outflow tract; Ao, aorta

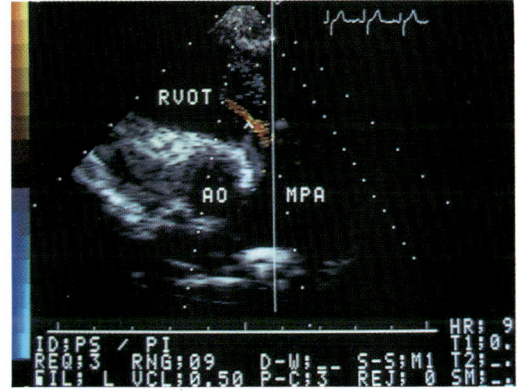

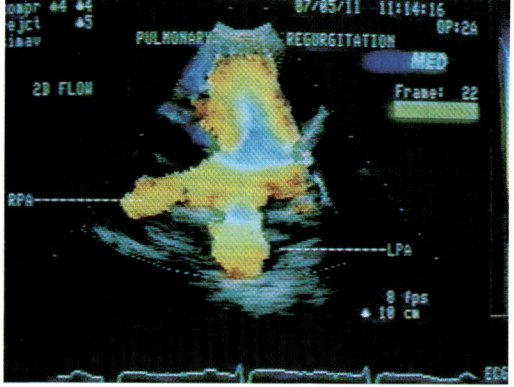

Plate 10 Colour Doppler recording for the child in *Figure 7.4* with severe pulmonary regurgitation. This diastolic frame shows retrograde flow in the pulmonary artery and extending into the branches.
RPA, right pulmonary artery; LPA, left pulmonary artery

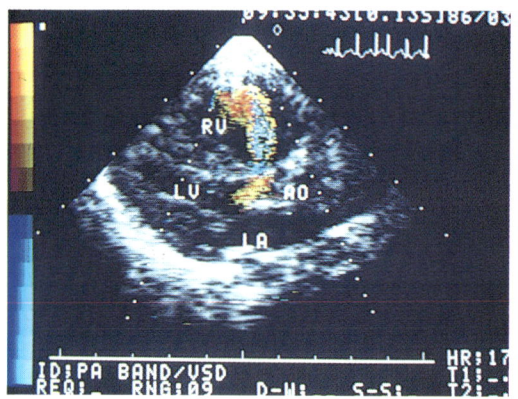

Plate 11 Parasternal long axis views in a patient with perimembranous ventricular septal defect showing (*a*) initial red flow as the blood passes superiorly towards the transducer from left ventricle (LV) to right ventricle (RV)

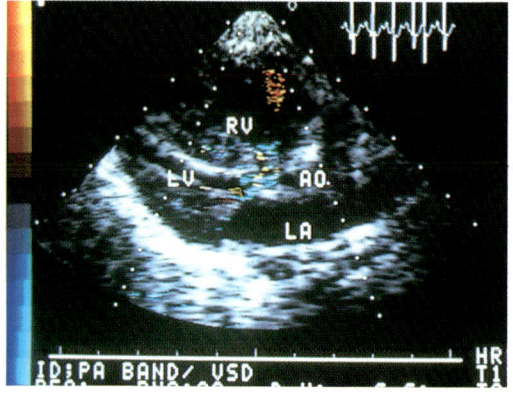

Plate 11 (*b*) at a slightly later time in systole, blue flow with flow reversal from right ventricle to left ventricular outflow tract. Ao, aorta; LA, left atrium

Plate 12 Colour Doppler flow mapping image in a patient with a small VSD which was not clearly demonstrated on echocardiogrpahy. The colour signal demonstrates its site in the muscular septum

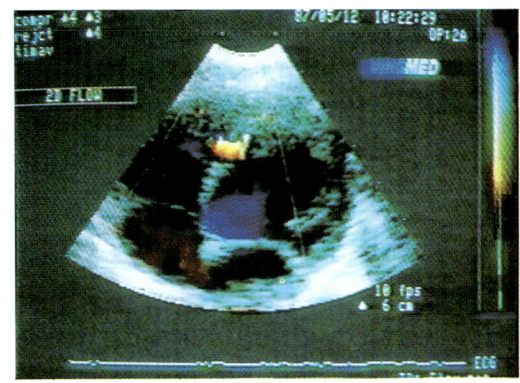

Plate 13 Long axis view from a man who received a stab injury 2 weeks before. The VSD in the muscular septum is shown by the flow through it; the lesion is a straight line which corresponds with the site of the skin laceration indicating a traumatic rather than congenital VSD

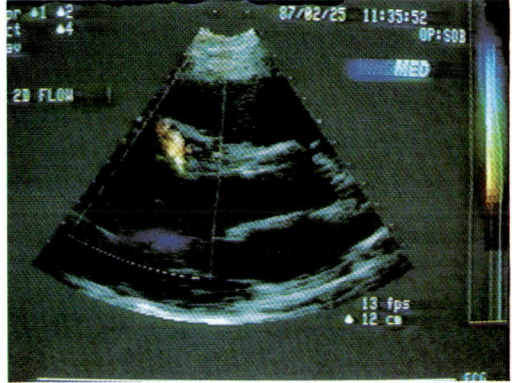

Plate 14 Parasternal short axis view demonstrating normal main pulmonary artery (MPA) flow in blue during systole with reversed flow arising at the head of the main pulmonary artery as flow enters from the patent ductus arteriosus (PDA) (arrows). This flow is confetti-like in appearance from turbulence and primarily left to right directed towards the transducer. Ao, aorta

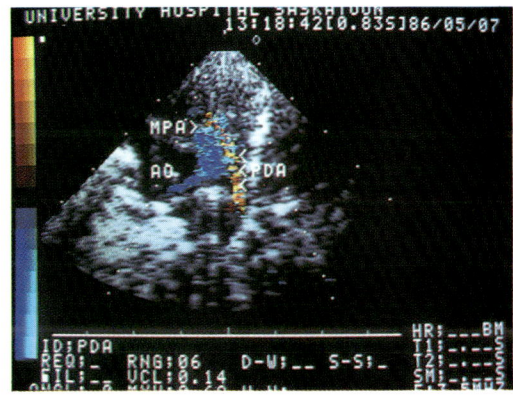

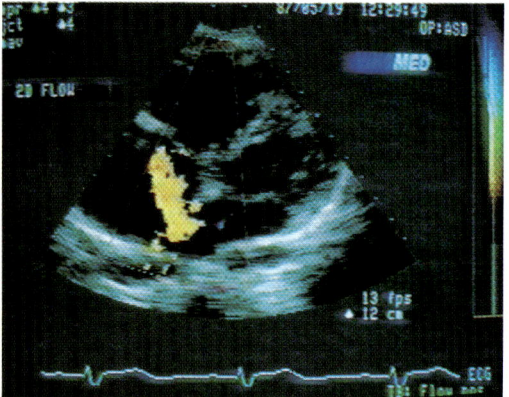

Plate 15 Colour Doppler flow mapping image showing flow through the atrial septum and thus outlining the margins of the defect

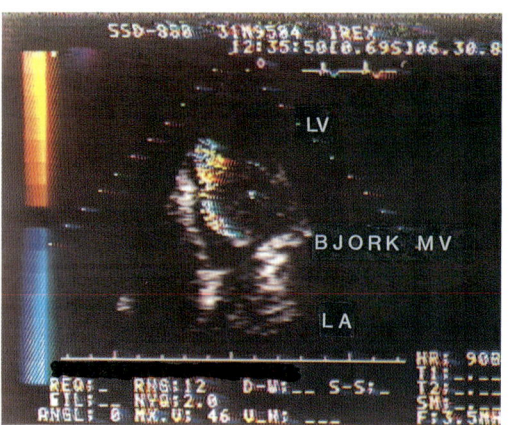

Plate 16 Colour Doppler flow map of patient with obstructed mitral prosthesis from the apical position. The high velocity aliased diastolic jet with a turbulent (mosaic) pattern is easily identified on the colour display. The origin at the orifice of the mitral prosthesis has a very narrow flow diameter which, in addition to the high velocity jet, indicates significant prosthetic valve obstruction

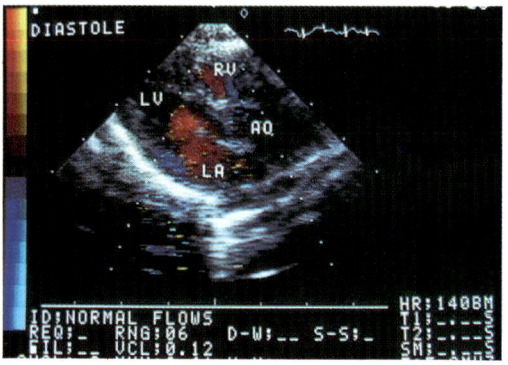

Plate 17 Parasternal long axis views demonstrating (*a*) diastolic mitral inflow in red as blood passes from left atrium (LA) to left ventricle (LV) with a small red blush in the right ventricle (RV) representing a small amount of the tricuspid inflow

Plate 17 Parasternal long axis views demonstrating (*b*) systolic egress of blood away from the left ventricle through the aortic root producing a blue image as flow passes away from the transducer. Ao, aorta

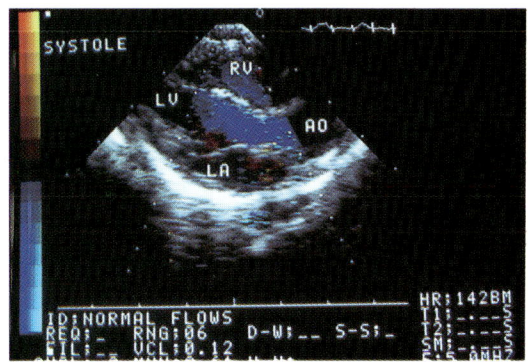

Plate 18 Parasternal short axis view at the level of the right ventricular outflow tract (RVOT), the main pulmonary artery and the pulmonary artery branches. Blood passing out of the right ventricle in this view is identified as blue and can be seen to divide into the two pulmonary artery branches. Ao, aorta; RPA, right pulmonary artery; LA, left pulmonary artery

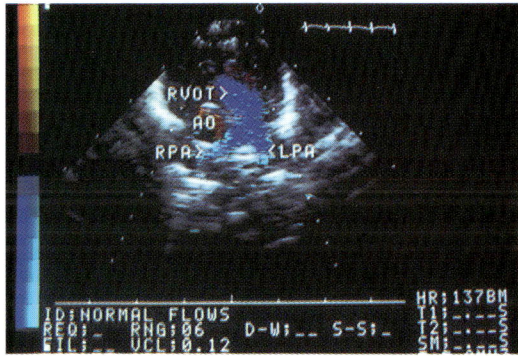

Plate 19 Apical four chamber view showing diastolic mitral and tricuspid inflow identified as red flow passing across the atrioventricular valves on either side of the interventricular septum (S). RV, right ventricle; RA, right atrium; LV, left ventricle; LA, left atrium

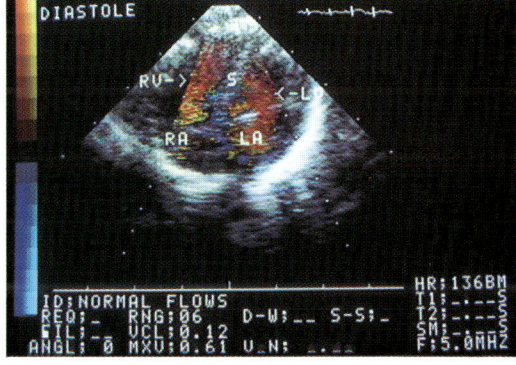

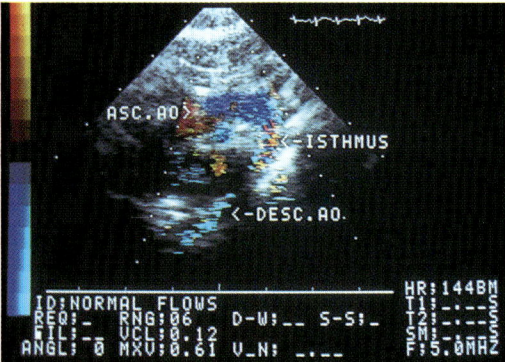

Plate 20 Suprasternal view of flow in the ascending aorta (ASC.Ao). Flow in the proximal ascending aorta is red (towards the transducer) and then becomes blue in colour as the flow passes around the aortic arch and into the descending aorta (DESC.Ao). In this particular study there was a mild flow turbulence in the region of the aortic isthmus producing a confetti-like appearance

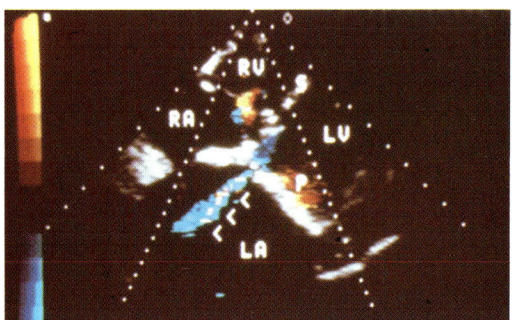

Plate 21 (*a*) Modified four chamber view performed intraoperatively. In the periprosthetic area, a high velocity blue jet was seen to be passing from the left ventricle (LV) to the left atrium (LA) (arrows)

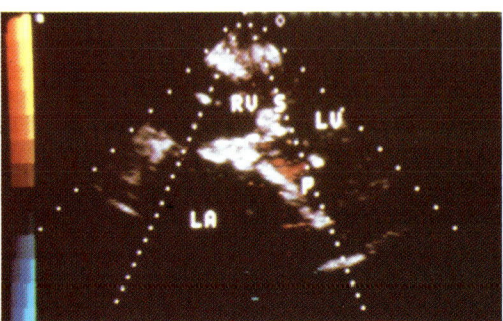

Plate 21 (*b*) Following repair of the ventriculo-atrial fistula the jet identifed in (*a*) has disappeared. RV, right ventricle; S, septum

unidentified by the peak-to-peak measurement performed at catheterization. However, although there may be a discrepancy in some patients with mild aortic stenosis this in no way affects the clinical value of the technique in predicting the need for surgical intervention, but one should have reservations about the accuracy of predicting aortic gradients in mild valvar obstruction. In these patients it is sensible to measure the flow velocity in the left ventricular outflow tract, proximal to the obstruction, and if an abnormally high velocity is present this proximal velocity should be included in the Bernoulli equation for more accurate estimation of the valve gradient.

If it is accepted that the severity of aortic stenosis can be assessed by non-invasive techniques the question of how this affects the need for cardiac catheterization has to be addressed. It can be argued that cardiac catheterization may be indicated for adults with valve lesions because of the possibility of coexistent ischaemic heart disease. Indeed, coronary angiography may well be indicated, but this is a much less hazardous and time consuming procedure than full right and left heart catheterization and in an appreciable number of patients undergoing catheterization for valvar disease coronary angiography is not even performed[3]. It would therefore seem safe and appropriate to recommend surgery in a number of patients with aortic stenosis without the need for prior cardiac catheterization. It is imperative however, that if clinical decisions are to be based on the information obtained by Doppler ultrasound, examination is performed by someone with considerable experience in Doppler ultrasound, in the full knowledge of the problems and pitfalls of the technique, with particular regard for the very real potential to underestimate significantly the aortic valve gradient in a patient with severe aortic stenosis.

Doppler is an extremely sensitive means of detecting aortic regurgitation, often demonstrating its presence in patients in whom it cannot be detected by clinical examination or other non-invasive tests. However, in this situation it is usually of no practical significance and its detection will not affect patient management. It would be very useful if Doppler could quantify the regurgitation but, although several techniques have been described, their exact value in assessing the situation either at a single time or on follow-up is still uncertain and any results must be interpreted with care. Thus a Doppler estimate of its severity can suggest whether it is of mild, moderate, or severe degree, but this is a rather crude assessment and similar to that on angiography. The decision on the need for surgical treatment is often not easy and the Doppler findings should be only one of the factors which must be taken into consideration.

Thus, combined methods of M-mode and two-dimensional echocardiography with pulsed, continuous wave and more recently two-dimensional Doppler colour flow mapping, can provide new and important methods for non-invasive assessment of aortic valve stenosis and regurgitation and it is likely that in the future it will be one of the most important techniques in determining the appropriate management of patients with aortic valve disease.

References

1. BLACKWOOD, R. A., BLOOM, K. R. and WILLIAMS, C. M. (1978) Aortic stenosis in children. Experience with prediction of severity. *Circulation,* **57,** 205–213
2. BRANDENBURG, R. O. (1981) No more routine catheterisation for valvular heart disease? (Editorial). *N. Eng. J. Med,* **305,** 1277–1278

3. HALL, R. J. C., KADUSHI, O. A. and EVEMY, K. (1983) Need for cardiac catheterisation in assessment of patients for valve surgery. *Br. Heart J.*, **49**, 268–275

4. HATLE, L. and ANGELSEN, B. (1985) *Doppler Ultrasound in Cardiology: Physical Principles and Clinical Applications*, 2nd edn, pp. 124–143. Philadelphia: Lea and Febiger

5. CURRIE, P. J., SEWARD, J. B., REEDER, G. S. *et al.* (1985) Continuous wave Doppler echocardiographic assessment of severity of calcific aortic stenosis: a simultaneous Doppler-catheter correlative study in 100 adult patients. *Circulation*, **71**, 1162–1169

6. CURRIE, P. J., HAGLER, D. J., SEWARD, J. B. *et al.* (1986) Instantaneous pressure gradient: a simultaneous Doppler and dual catheter correlative study. *J. Am. Coll. Cardiol.*, **7**, 800–806

7. ZHANG, Y., MYHRE, E. and NITTER-HAUGE, S. (1985) Noninvasive quantification of the aortic valve area in aortic stenosis by Doppler echocardiography. *Eur. Heart J.*, **6**, 992–998

8. CALLAHAN, M. J., TAJIK, A. J., SU-FAN, Q. and BOVE, A. (1985) Validation of instantaneous pressure gradients measured by continuous wave Doppler in experimentally induced aortic stenosis. *Am. J. Cardiol.*, **56**, 989–993

9. SMITH, M. D., DAWSON, P. L., ELION, J. L. *et al.* (1985) Correlation of continuous wave Doppler velocities with cardiac catheterisation gradients: an experimental model of aortic stenosis. *J. Am. Coll. Cardiol.*, **6**, 1306–1314

10. OHLSSON, J. and WRANNE, B. (1986) Noninvasive assessment of valve area in patients with aortic stenosis. *J. Am. Coll. Cardiol.*, **7**, 501–508

11. TEIRSTEIN, P., YEAGER, M., YOCK, P. G. and POPP, R. L. (1986) Doppler echocardiographic measurement of aortic valve area in aortic stenosis: a noninvasive application of the Gorlin formula. *J. Am. Coll. Cardiol.*, **8**, 1059–1065

12. OTTO, C. M., PEARLMAN, A. S., COMESS, K. A., REAMER, R. P., JANKO, C. L. and HUNTSMAN, L. L. (1986) Determination of the stenotic aortic valve area in adults using Doppler echocardiography. *J. Am. Coll. Cardiol.*, **7**, 509–517

13. SKJAERPE, T., HEGRENAES, L. and HATLE, L. (1985) Noninvasive estimation of valve area in patients with aortic stenosis by Doppler ultrasound and two-dimensional echocardiography. *Circulation*, **72**, 810–818

14. TOUCHE, T., PRASQUIER, R., NITENBERG, A., DE ZUTTERE, D. and GOURGON, R. (1985) Assessment and follow-up of patients with aortic regurgitation by an updated Doppler echocardiographic measurement of the regurgitant fraction in the aortic arch. *Circulation*, **72**, 819–824

15. KITABATAKE, A., ITO, H., INOUE, M. *et al.* (1985) A new approach to noninvasive evaluation of aortic regurgitation fraction by two-dimensional Doppler echocardiography. *Circulation*, **72**, 523–529

16. SIMPSON, I. A., HOUSTON, A. B., SHELDON, C. S., HUTTON, I. and LAWRIE, T. D. V. (1985) Clinical value of Doppler echocardiography in the assessment of adults with aortic stenosis. *Br. Heart J.*, **53**, 636–639

5

Mitral valve disease

A. P. G. Mayala and J. Roelandt

The investigation and management of patients with mitral valve disease remains a common problem in adult cardiology, particularly in the parts of the world where acute rheumatic fever is still common. The mitral valve can be affected in a variety of ways. In mitral stenosis, which is commonly the result of rheumatic fever, the leaflets are predominantly involved. Mitral valve regurgitation may result from dysfunction or destruction of any component of the valve apparatus, including on occasions abnormalities of segmental contraction produced by ischaemia (coronary artery disease) or altered geometry (cardiomyopathy, heart failure).

Surgical recommendations in these patients are solidly based on symptoms and clinical examination. Further investigations are directed at confirming the diagnosis and providing anatomical and functional information. The severity of mitral stenosis can usually be assessed accurately by clinical examination, electrocardiography (ECG), and chest X-ray. Two-dimensional echocardiography can then provide the necessary anatomical information, namely left atrial size, mitral valve area and the presence of calcification. However, difficulties can arise where other valve lesions coexist or where clinical signs and symptoms are complicated by the presence of pulmonary disease and cardiac catheterization may then be necessary. Furthermore, since the information it provides is largely anatomical, it is less accurate in the assessment of mitral regurgitation and where stenosis and regurgitation coexist the relative contribution of each lesion to the patient's problem may not always be readily apparent.

Thus, echocardiography can only give indirect evidence of the haemodynamic effects of mitral valve function. Doppler ultrasound has the potential to enhance non-invasive diagnosis in these patients by the addition of this important haemodynamic information. It now permits a quantitative assessment of transmitral blood flow and measurement of blood flow velocity across a stenotic or leaking mitral valve, thus providing a means to calculate the pressure drop and valve orifice area[1–4]. Colour Doppler flow mapping may further expand the clinical usefulness of echo/Doppler for the analysis of the mitral valve, particularly in the presence of multivalvar disease, and for the evaluation of regurgitation.

The clinical impact of Doppler ultrasound in patients with mitral valve disease, particularly mitral stenosis, may be less than for other lesions because of the accuracy of clinical and current non-invasive investigations. However, the information Doppler provides is both confirmatory and complementary to these established techniques and can only further enhance the accuracy of the non-invasive assessment of patients with mitral valve disease.

Examination technique

There will be minor variations in the examination technique depending on the Doppler instrumentation used for measuring the mitral valve flow velocity. It is similar to that described for measuring normal mitral flow in Chapter 3.

The examination is best performed with the patient in the left lateral decubitus position. The mitral flow is most easily obtained with the transducer positioned for long axis and four chamber views and tilted until maximum Doppler shifts are obtained. For conventional Doppler with an integrated ultrasound imaging system, cross-sectional views and thus anatomical landmarks are used for orientation for Doppler interrogation. In Doppler systems without imaging capabilities, the audio and spectral signals are used for orientation; this procedure can be time consuming and tedious, but after some experience good quality recordings can be obtained in most patients. Colour Doppler flow mapping overcomes most of the practical limitations of conventional Doppler techniques[5, 6]. It allows real-time visualization of both spatially correlated normal and abnormal transmitral blood flow velocities and their dispersion and superimposes them on cross-sectional images using colour-coded flow schemes (*see Plate 2*).

In order accurately to obtain the pressure drop across an obstructed mitral valve, it is important to record the instantaneous maximal velocities. The sampling site influences the Doppler signal and different apical and parasternal positions should be explored to obtain the maximal velocity signal, thus ensuring optimal alignment of the beam to the jet. The use of an integrated imaging system to give cross-sectional views and thus anatomical landmarks for orientation for Doppler interrogation does not always improve the recording of maximal velocities due to the variability in direction of blood flow relative to the anatomical landmarks and it is worthwhile trying to obtain a higher velocity without imaging. Potentially improper alignment of the interrogating Doppler beam may cause underestimation of velocities and pressure drops[2, 3], although colour Doppler flow mapping may help to overcome this problem and improve the diagnostic accuracy.

When using pulsed Doppler the sample volume can be sited with precision, but with diseased valves there is the obvious limitation of the relatively low maximal velocity which can be measured without the aliasing phenomenon occurring[7]. The possibility of aliasing increases with depth and with higher blood flow velocities and is relatively common in large patients with mitral stenosis. The aliasing problem may be reduced by decreasing the depth of the sample volume (by choosing a different transducer location on the chest), by using the zero-shift technique, or by switching to high pulse repetition frequency or continuous wave Doppler. The pulsed Doppler mode offers the advantage that it permits range resolution so that flow can be characterized in any selected location along the sound beam axis. On the other hand, with the continuous wave mode very high velocities can be measured but there is no range resolution. Since assessment of the mitral valve requires measurement of the highest velocities which only occur in the area of interest (i.e. in the defect), range resolution is not a necessity and the continuous wave modality is most commonly used for the study of mitral valve disease.

With colour Doppler flow mapping the problem of aliasing occurs for the same physical reasons. Thus velocities exceeding the Nyquist limit for a given pulse repetition frequency are encoded with the reversed colour which gives an artefactual impression of flow reversal on the display (*see Plate 2*). However, the aliasing phenomenon in colour Doppler indicates the site and direction of the

the maximum velocities and facilitates the interrogation of such high velocity jets by continuous wave Doppler allowing optimal alignment of the jet flow and sound beam or the accurate determination of the angle between the two.

Normal transmitral flow velocity pattern

In normal subjects the mitral flow waveform can be measured with the pulsed technique: passive transmitral flow begins with the opening of the mitral valve, rapidly reaches a maximum, then diminishes (and may fall to zero when diastole is long) until late diastole when it again increases with atrial contraction and ceases with the closure of the mitral valve (*Figure 5.1*). This Doppler velocity trace reflects pressure differences between the left atrium and left ventricle and transmitral volume flow. The normal peak transmitral blood velocity is seldom above 1.0 m/s, but values up to 1.3 m/s can be obtained. Normally no systolic flow signal is detected.

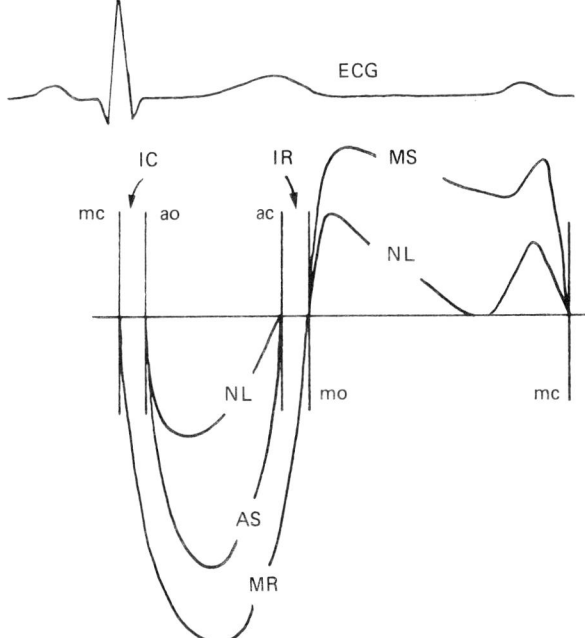

Figure 5.1 Diagrammatic summary of the normal maximal Doppler velocity waveform (NL) and those in various left heart conditions. The normal velocity waveform can be recorded with the pulsed Doppler technique but pathological conditions will require continuous wave Doppler interrogation because of increased velocities exceeding the Nyquist limit. Normal passive transmitral inflow begins with the opening of the mitral valve (mo) and is completed before the active phase begins. The active phase, produced by atrial contraction, terminates with mitral valve closure (mc). Peak velocities are seldom above 1 m/s. In mitral stenosis (MS) blood flow velocities are higher and the passive inflow phase extends throughout diastole in diminishing magnitude. The velocity contour follows the pressure gradient. The increase in velocities which results from atrial contraction is missing when atrial fibrillation is present. In mitral regurgitation (MR) velocities begin with the closure of the mitral valve (mc) and their peak takes a rounded form in mid-systole extending throughout systole and ending with mitral valve opening (mo). In aortic stenosis (AS) a pattern similar to that of mitral regurgitation is recorded but the flow duration starting with the aortic valve opening (ao) and ending with the aortic valve closure (ac) is shorter than that of mitral regurgitation. Consideration of valve movements is therefore useful for their differentiation. ECG: electrocardiogram, IC: isovolumic contraction phase, IR: isovolumic relaxation phase

Mitral stenosis

Doppler echocardiography has dramatically improved our ability to quantify mitral valve disease by non-invasive means. With the Doppler technique it is possible to study the blood velocity pattern across the obstructed mitral valve and from the maximum velocity tracings to calculate transmitral pressure drops using the modified Bernoulli equation:

$$P1 - P2 = 4V^2$$

where P1 is the atrial pressure, P2 is the pressure in the mitral orifice and V the maximal recorded velocity[1, 8].

In patients with mitral stenosis the most characteristic change is the increased maximum blood flow velocity (usually exceeding 1.5 m/s), with the passive inflow phase extending throughout diastole and exhibiting a gradual slow decrease in velocity, in contrast to the rapid decrease in normal subjects (*Figures 5.1, 5.2* and *5.3*). The increase in velocities which results from atrial contraction is absent when atrial fibrillation is present. Using colour flow Doppler mapping the stenotic inflow jet is readily visualized and has a 'flame-shaped' appearance due to central aliasing and peripheral turbulence. Guided interrogation of the jet with optimal alignment of the jet flow and sound beam allows determination of the angle between the two and hence a more accurate velocity measurement in some patients (*see Plate 3*).

In several studies a moderately good correlation has been demonstrated between Doppler measurements of pressure drop and simultaneous pressure recordings during cardiac catheterization[1, 2]. It is important to realize, however, that the estimation of the pressure drop across a stenotic valve by the Doppler technique with the use of the Bernoulli equation is not directly comparable with an invasive catheter pressure drop measurement. Energy losses at the inlet of the stenotic mitral valve, non-uniformity of velocity distribution and pressure recovery component in the outlet region limit the accuracy and comparison between Doppler and catheter pressure drop measurements.

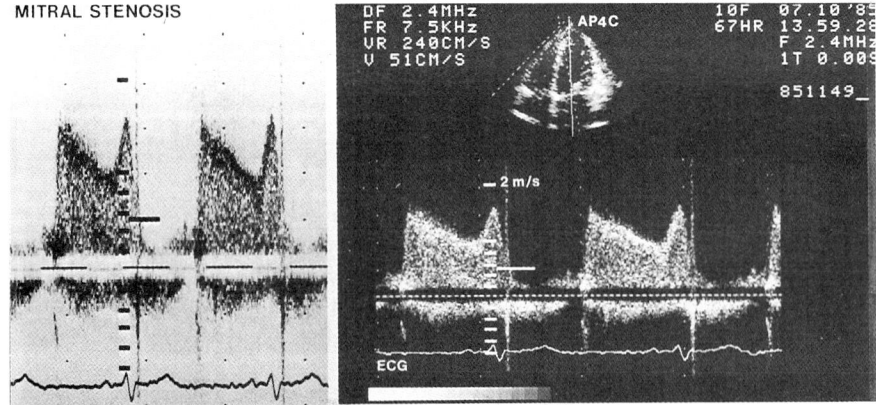

Figure 5.2 Blood flow velocity over the mitral valve sampled from the apical transducer position in the four chamber view (AP4C) in a patient with mild mitral stenosis and sinus rhythm. The initial velocity is increased (1.5 m/s) and the typical 'M' configuration apparent. The second peak velocity at end-diastole results from atrial contraction. ECG, electrocardiogram

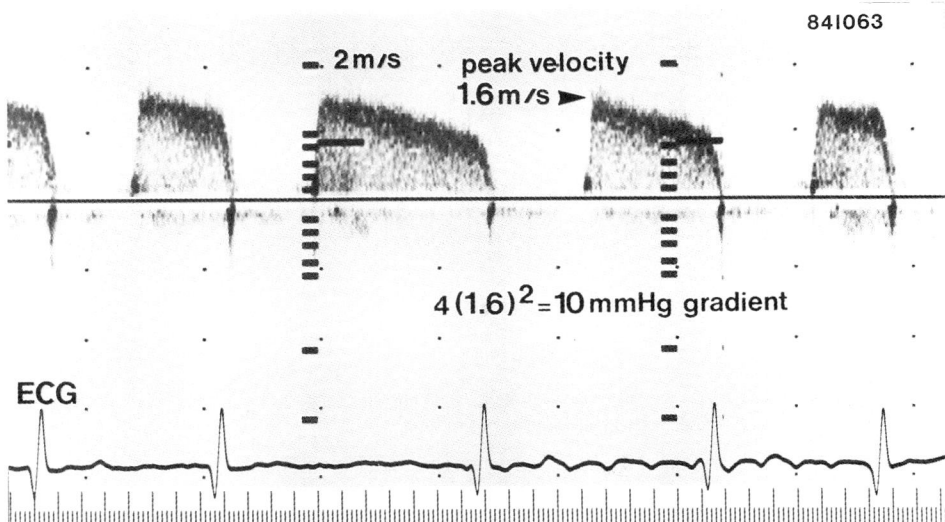

Figure 5.3 Pulsed Doppler tracing from a patient with mild to moderate mitral stenosis. The early diastolic velocity reaches 1.6 m/s corresponding to a pressure drop of 10 mmHg. There is a slow decline in diastolic velocities as a result of the reduced rate of pressure equalization between left atrium and left ventricle representing reduced emptying of the left atrium. There is no late diastolic increase of velocity because the patient is in atrial fibrillation

In clinical terms, the peak mitral gradient is of little relevance as mitral gradients at catheterization are usually measured as a mean value over the diastolic time period. Calculation of the peak pressure drop from the peak mitral flow velocity will not therefore relate to a mean gradient as measured at catheterization and the mean pressure drop across the mitral valve should therefore be calculated to provide meaningful information about the severity of mitral stenosis. Since the relationship between velocity and pressure drop is not linear, averaging the maximum velocity over diastole and applying the modified Bernoulli equation is not valid. The instantaneous pressure drop must be calculated from the maximum velocity at each point throughout diastole, for practical purposes at each 5 or 10 ms interval and then averaged to estimate the mean gradient. In practical terms this requires a computer-aided analysis system, but since the software for making this measurement is available in most commercial Doppler machines it is easily performed. The line of the maximum velocity is traced manually or electronically and the computer simply instructed to calculate the mean gradient; to increase the reliability of the calculation it is necessary to trace 10 consecutive beats in patients in sinus rhythm and 15 beats in those in atrial fibrillation. This method is well suited for both the diagnosis and the follow-up of patients with mitral stenosis but suffers from the disadvantage that the value can vary with flow across the valve and heart rate.

Most invasive studies include calculation of mitral valve orifice area to determine the severity of mitral stenosis. However, it has also been suggested that an assessment of severity of mitral stenosis can be made by the use of the pressure half-time, which represents the time interval during which the pressure difference falls to half of its initial maximum value in early diastole[9]. Doppler velocity tracings can also be used for the calculation of pressure half-time[2, 8]: the early

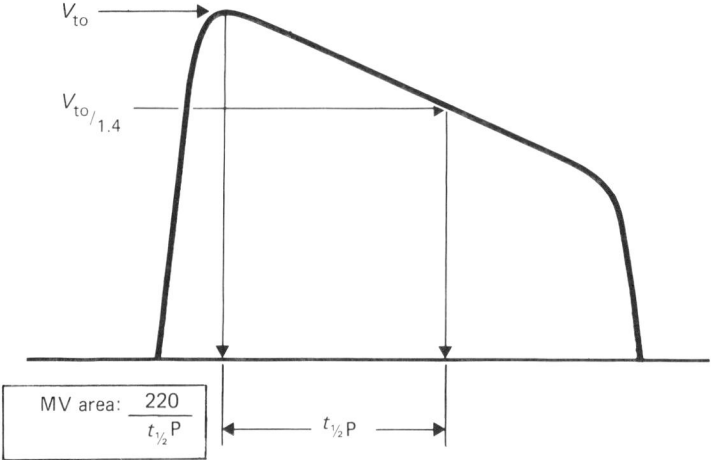

Figure 5.4 The principle of measuring transmitral pressure half-time and calculating mitral valve orifice area from Doppler. The initial or early diastolic velocity (V_{to}) is measured and corresponds to a pressure drop of $4V_{to}^2$. Half this pressure is thus $4V_{to}^2/2$. This equation can be rearranged such that the velocity which represents this pressure is $V_{to}/\sqrt{2}$. Thus the velocity equivalent to the pressure half-time is obtained by dividing the initial peak velocity (V_{to}) by the square root of 2 (i.e. 1.4). Once this value has been calculated, the point at which the mitral velocity decreases to this value is located. The time between V_{to} and $V_{to}/1.4$ is the transmitral pressure half-time ($t_{1/2}p$). The $t_{1/2}p$ is inversely proportional to the mitral valve orifice area. By dividing 220 (an empirically derived constant) by $t_{1/2}p$ (in ms), the mitral valve orifice area in cm^2 can be obtained

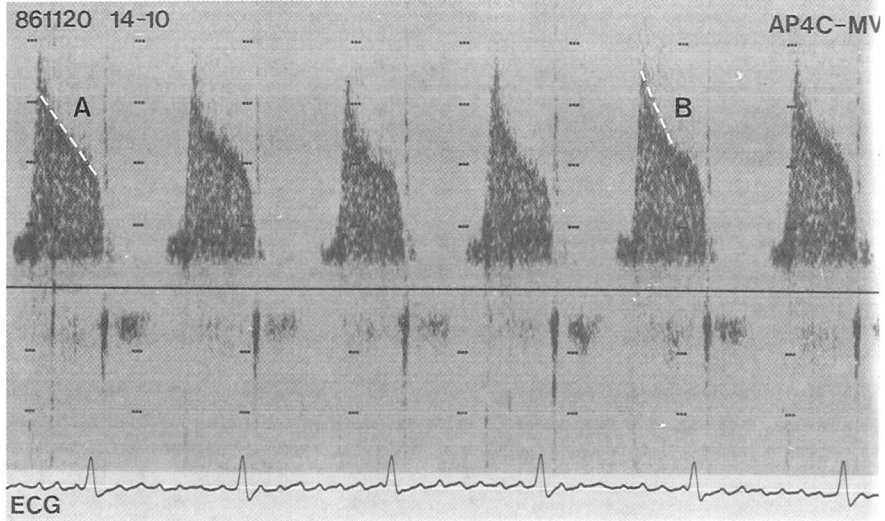

Figure 5.5 Blood flow velocity of the mitral valve from the apical transducer position in a patient with mitral stenosis. The signal exhibits an early diastolic short high peak velocity. There are two possibilities for measurement of transmitral pressure half-time from such recordings. A: ignore the early high peak velocity and use the linear part of the curve. Pressure half-time is then 197 ms. B: use the slope of the sharp velocity peak. Pressure half-time is 87 ms. At our institution we ignore the early peak velocity and use measurement A. Because of the measurement variability at least 10 consecutive beats are analysed and the mean $t_{1/2}p$ used for valve area calculation, ECG, electrocardiogram

maximal diastolic velocity is divided by 1.4 (the square root of 2) to give the velocity corresponding to half that maximal pressure value; the time from the initial peak to the point on the curve at which this pressure occurs then represents the pressure half-time (*Figure 5.4*). A number of cycles should be averaged, as for the mean pressure calculation. The mitral pressure half-time in a normal individual is less than 60 ms and in those with mitral stenosis above 100 ms, the time increasing progressively with decrease in valve area.

Mitral valve area can then be estimated by dividing 220 (an empirically derived constant) by the pressure half-time expressed in milliseconds. Thus a pressure half-time of 220 ms predicts a mitral valve area of 1.0 cm^2. The value is thought to be relatively independent of mitral flow and heart rate. The mitral valve area calculated non-invasively correlates well with that obtained from catheterization data[3]. There may be practical problems, however, in deriving pressure half-time in patients who have a non-linear decay in velocity. When there is a short sharp peak in early diastole, most often representing a valve artefact, this part can be disregarded in the analysis (*Figure 5.5*).

Mitral regurgitation

Doppler ultrasound can diagnose a mitral regurgitant lesion by the demonstration of systolic retrograde flow through or adjacent to the mitral valve and passing into the left atrial cavity.

The signal is of relatively high velocity and continuous wave Doppler is necessary to demonstrate the full waveform. The classical continuous wave signal shows that the velocities begin with the closure of the mitral valve, extend throughout systole with the peak taking a rounded form in mid-systole, end with mitral valve opening, and may continue as the positive forward diastolic flow (*see Figure 5.1*). With pulsed Doppler the signal can be tracked back from the ventricle to the atrium: recording in the left ventricle shows only forward diastolic mitral flow, at the orifice both forward and regurgitant flow are recorded, in the atrium mainly regurgitant flow is found. The systolic jet of mitral regurgitation should be sought by Doppler interrogation from both the parasternal and apical transducer positions because the regurgitant jet may not be found if it is directed out of the plane of any single two-dimensional view. Indeed, the use of the image can be misleading and it is often easier to search for this signal with a non-imaging transducer since the jet may be at an unexpected angle to the valve as seen on the echocardiogram. The regurgitant signal will not necessarily be obtained from the position giving the best diastolic one. With the colour Doppler flow mapping technique it is possible to visualize a regurgitant jet that is apparently in a direction opposite to that which is expected at a given point in the cardiac cycle. Because of the high velocity and turbulence aliasing occurs which results in a mosaic of colours (*see Plates 4* and *5*). The method greatly facilitates the diagnosis and may help to grade semiquantitatively the severity of valvar insufficiency[6, 10].

Doppler is an extremely sensitive technique and may even demonstrate lesions which are not apparent clinically. On the other hand, regurgitation can be missed if the jet is in an unusual line and sufficient care is not taken in seeking it. However, Doppler would be more useful in mitral regurgitation if it could quantify the degree of regurgitation and assess the severity of the lesion. The quantitative accuracy of the Doppler method is difficult to evaluate due to the limited accuracy of the reference methods.

Mapping-techniques, where a range-gated sample volume is moved around the left atrial cavity, have been proposed to assess the severity of the regurgitation by measuring the breadth and extent of the jet[11, 12]. This approach is a blind technique and therefore cumbersome and time consuming. Moreover, regurgitant jets may be eccentric especially in mitral valve prolapse or a leaking prosthetic valve and part of it is easily missed. The sample volume may also overlap in a contiguous chamber and detect potentially misleading flows such as in the aorta when one searches for an eccentric regurgitant jet in the left atrium. It might be expected that colour Doppler will give a clearer demonstration of the extent of backflow. A good agreement between the planimetered surface area of the jet and the cineangiographic assessment of severity of mitral regurgitation has been reported[10], but this has not been a universal finding.

Apart from experience in using the technique there are several factors to explain this discrepancy. First, there are fundamental differences between the topographic display of the velocities of a regurgitant jet by Doppler and its densitographic display by angiocardiography after the injection of a radiopaque contact medium. Second, the length, area and timing of a regurgitant jet are not only related to the site of the defect but also to the pressure drop across the valve and the compliance of the receiving chamber. An important yet unknown factor in any given patient is the irregular shape of the defect which will cause turbulence, leading to a loss of kinetic energy and decrease in the length/area of the jet. The colour coding and thus the display of the surface area of a regurgitant jet may also be affected by technical factors, in particular the signal-to-noise ratio and characteristics of the high pass filter. Thus despite initial great and widespread enthusiasm, quantification of regurgitant lesions is only semiquantitative at best and a close agreement with angiocardiography must not be expected.

It has been suggested that it is possible to quantitate the regurgitant volume by subtracting the stroke volume through another competent valve from that through

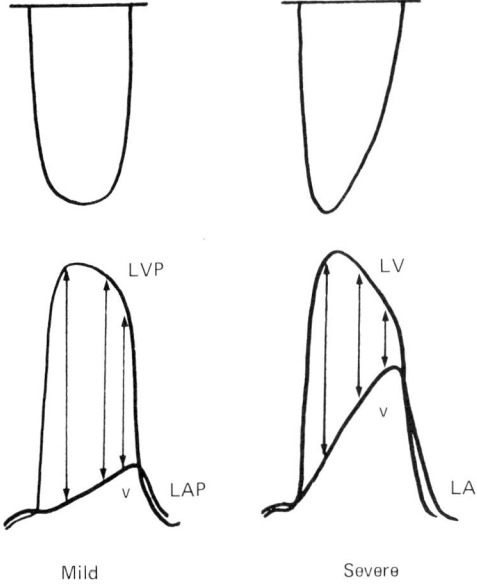

Figure 5.6 Doppler flow patterns in mitral regurgitation. In mild to moderate regurgitation the pressure stays high in the left ventricle (LVP) and low in the left atrium (LAP) whereby the LV-LA pressure difference remains high during systole, resulting in high velocity difference throughout systole. With severe regurgitation the LV pressure falls more rapidly and the LA pressure increases dramatically, resulting in a prominent V-wave. The LV-LA pressure difference decreases quickly resulting in a diminished velocity

the regurgitant one. The limitation of this method is the inaccuracy of the stroke volume estimation with possible inaccuracies being doubled by making the measurement at two sites.

Using continuous wave Doppler some qualitative assessment of severity can be obtained from the intensity of the regurgitant signal since this is related to the volume of blood travelling at that particular velocity within the Doppler sample beam. Furthermore, since forward flow through the mitral valve will be increased in significant regurgitation, confirmation of severe mitral regurgitation may be obtained from an increase in the peak mitral diastolic velocity to greater than 2.0 m/s which is outside the range of normality. The presence of mitral stenosis will invalidate this and it should therefore be ignored in the absence of a normal pressure half-time.

Some idea of the severity of the regurgitation can be obtained from the waveform of the maximal blood flow velocities during systole (*Figure 5.6, 5.7* and *5.8; see Plate 4*). Continuous wave Doppler is needed to record the high velocities producing the signal. In mild to moderately severe regurgitation the pressure remains high in the left ventricle and low in the left atrium with the result that, throughout systole, both the pressure difference and the Doppler velocity remain high. In severe (volume) regurgitation the ventricular pressure falls more rapidly and the atrial pressure increases dramatically, resulting in a prominent V-wave. The pressure difference decreases rapidly resulting in a rapidly diminishing blood flow velocity (*see Plate 4*). Thus, these blood flow velocity patterns can give an idea of the severity of the regurgitation.

A practical problem can often occur when mitral regurgitation coexists with aortic stenosis and, particularly with a non-imaging system, it is difficult to decide which of these causes the high velocity systolic signal. The onset and termination of

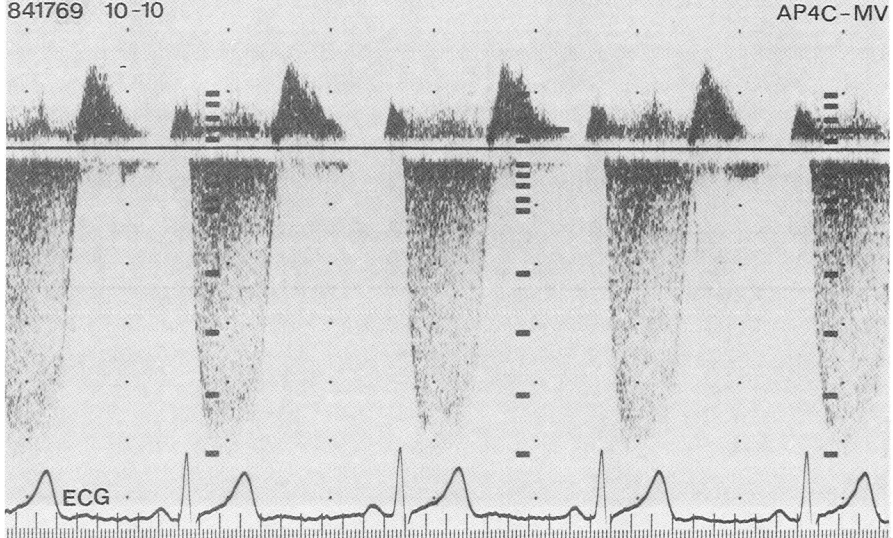

Figure 5.7 Continuous wave Doppler blood flow velocity recording of a patient with moderate to mild mitral regurgitation. The systolic blood flow velocity has a fast rate of rise and the velocity remains high throughout systole corresponding to a mild to moderate volume regurgitation

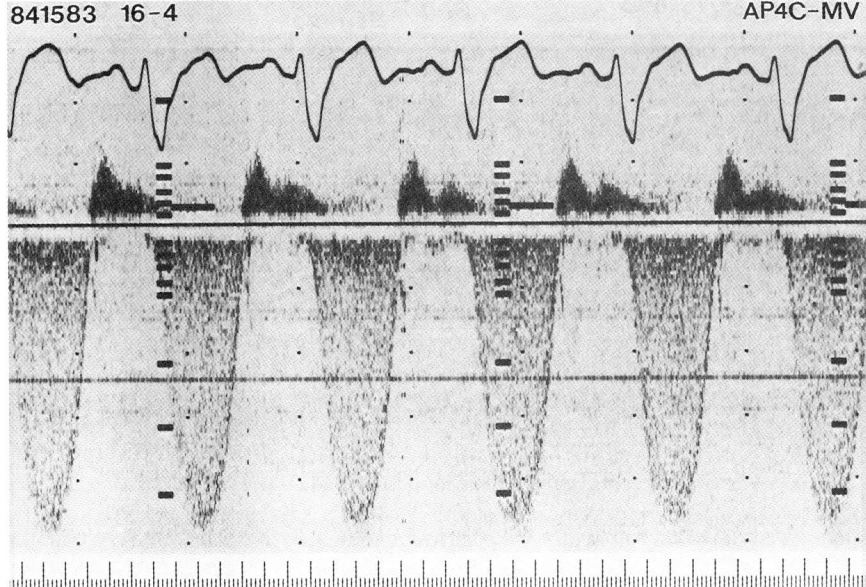

841583   16-4   AP4C-MV

Figure 5.8 Doppler flow velocity recording of a patient with poor left ventricular function and moderate to severe mitral regurgitation recorded from the apical transducer position with continuous wave Doppler. The maximal velocity is approximately 4.5 m/s indicating a LV-LA pressure difference of about 80 mmHg. The slow rate of rise of the blood velocity curve indicates poor left ventricular function (equivalent of low dp/dt). The rapid fall of velocities is consistent with a moderate to large volume regurgitation

the regurgitant velocity trace is helpful in this differentiation (*see Figure 5.1*): the mitral signal is of longer duration, continuing from closure to opening of the mitral valve, while the shorter aortic signal lasts from opening to closure of its valve. Colour Doppler imaging is particularly helpful in this situation.

Clinical application of Doppler ultrasound

Mitral stenosis, the most common sequel to rheumatic fever, has become less common in developed parts of the world, but still presents a major problem in certain areas, which are precisely those where elaborate invasive facilities are scarce. In most cases the diagnosis can be made and the severity assessed by the accepted non-invasive techniques, in particular echocardiography, such that catheterization is not generally required. However, further confirmatory evidence is always of value, in particular if it allows quantitation of the severity which is useful not only for diagnosis but also for serial follow-up. The assessment of mitral stenosis is one of the easiest applications of the technique with good quality recordings being obtained from the apex in virtually all patients. Thus one of the most important clinical applications of Doppler echocardiography involves the determination of pressure drop and the calculation of mitral valve area in mitral stenosis.

The accuracy of Doppler ultrasound measurements of pressure drops and valve areas has been confirmed by much experience, and validation of the simplified Bernoulli equation both *in vivo* and *in vitro*[13] has found that Doppler ultrasound does accurately estimate the pressure drop across a wide variety of clinically encountered obstructions to blood flow.

In clinical practice, in adults with mitral stenosis a continuous wave signal is likely to be necessary for determining the severity. The maximum velocity is of little practical value but, if the equipment allows this to be performed easily, the mean pressure drop is worth calculating since it provides a value comparable to that routinely measured at catheterization with which physicians and surgeons are familiar. However, this measurement is dependent on transvalvar flow and heart rate and a value obtained at an outpatient visit will not be comparable to that from the catheterization laboratory with the patient sedated, as discussed in Chapter 4. It is, therefore, more useful to measure the pressure half-time and, if necessary for those not familiar with this technique, present the result as the valve area. These values do vary with rate, activity and flow but much less than the gradient and will still provide a useful assessment even in the presence of mitral regurgitation or poor ventricular function.

Doppler presents an extremely sensitive means for diagnosing mitral regurgitation, so much so that lesions not apparent on clinical examination can often be easily detected. This is of little practical value and it would be more important to be able to assess the severity of regurgitation. The quantitation of regurgitant volume is so fraught with possible inaccuracies that its measurement is probably worthless in practical terms, except in a research capacity. An idea whether the regurgitation is mild, moderate or severe is obtained by assessing the extent of the regurgitant flow with either conventional pulsed or colour flow mapping. This is also subject to errors in performance and interpretation and does not give an exact comparison with ventriculography. It must also be remembered that a regurgitant jet at an unusual angle may be missed by Doppler. The technique may be of little help in deciding on the need for surgery in any particular patient, but early and rapid fall in the velocity of the jet will indicate a high left atrial pressure, and where possible measurement of the velocity of pulmonary or tricuspid regurgitation will allow a prediction of the pulmonary artery pressure (*see* Chapters 6 and 7).

Doppler may be of particular use in the assessment of multivalve disease where the individual contribution of the aortic or mitral lesion to the patient's symptoms is uncertain. Under these circumstances the differentiation between a high-velocity jet produced by aortic stenosis and that produced by mitral regurgitation may be difficult; careful study of the duration of flow in relation to valve movements should show that the duration of mitral regurgitation is longer than that of aortic flow. These problems can, however, be overcome by using colour Doppler flow mapping, which enables direct visualization of a regurgitant or stenotic jet. Mitral regurgitation is easily diagnosed and grading of the severity can be performed semiquantitatively based on the farthest distance reached and the area covered by the regurgitant jet flow. The technique also offers advantages for the diagnosis of multivalvar heart disease where clinical differentiation may be difficult and conventional pulsed Doppler findings confusing. An example is mixed mitral stenosis and aortic insufficiency where two jet flows overlap each other. Here one lesion may be overestimated or the second lesion may be missed. In addition, eccentric jets may be difficult to assess with conventional pulsed Doppler and are now readily visualized.

Thus Doppler provides accurate diagnosis and quantitative assessment of the severity of mitral stenosis. It is a very sensitive and specific method for the detection of mitral regurgitation and gives a semiquantitative assessment of its severity. It may be considered that Doppler has limited clinical value in this context because echocardiography is very accurate for mitral stenosis and, since mitral regurgitation is usually apparent clinically, its detection is not of major clinical importance. However, these applications complement M-mode and two-dimensional echocardiography in mitral disease and can provide confirmatory and additional information allowing a more confident recommendation of surgical intervention, where necessary, without catheterization. This may have particular relevance as a screening and diagnostic procedure in countries where rheumatic heart disease is common and patient numbers are large but facilities limited.

References

1. HOLEN, J., AASLID, R., LANDMARK, K. and SIMONSEN, S. (1976) Determination of pressure gradient in mitral stenosis with a non-invasive ultrasound Doppler technique. *Acta Med. Scand.*, **199**, 455–460
2. HATLE, L., BRUBAKK, A., TROMSDAL, A. and ANGELSEN, B. (1978) Non-invasive assessment of pressure drop in mitral stenosis by Doppler ultrasound. *Br. Heart J.*, **40**, 131–140
3. HATLE, L., ANGELSEN, B. and TROMSDAL, A. (1979) Non-invasive assessment of atrioventricular pressure half time by Doppler ultrasound. *Circulation*, **60**, 1096–1104
4. REQUARTH, J. A., GOLDBERG, S. J., VASKO, S. D. and ALLEN, H. D. (1984) *In vitro* verification of Doppler prediction of transvalve pressure gradient and orifice area in stenosis. *Am. J. Cardiol.*, **52**, 1369–1373
5. ROELANDT, J. (1986) Colour-coded Doppler flow imaging: what are the prospects? *Eur. Heart J.*, **7**, 184
6. MIYATAKE, K., OKAMOTO, M., KINOSHITA, N. *et al.* (1984) Clinical application of a new type of real-time two-dimensional flow imaging system. *Am. J. Cardiol.*, **54**, 857–868
7. BOM, N., DE BOO, J. and RIJSTERBORGH, H. (1984) On the aliasing problem in pulsed Doppler cardiac studies. *J. Clin. Ultrasound*, **12**, 559–567
8. HATLE, L. and ANGELSEN, B. (1985) *Doppler Ultrasound in Cardiology: Physical Principles and Clinical Applications*, 2nd edn., pp. 110–124. Philadelphia: Lea & Febiger
9. LIBANOFF, A. J. and RODBARD, S. (1968) Atrioventricular pressure half-time: measurement of mitral valve orifice area. *Circulation*, **38**, 44–50
10. OMOTO, R., YOKOTE, Y., TAKAMOTO, S. *et al.* (1984) The development of real-time two-dimensional Doppler echocardiography and its clinical significance in acquired valvular disease: with specific reference to the evaluation of valvular regurgitation. *Jpn. Heart J.*, **25**, 325–340
11. ABBASI, A. S., ALLEN, M. W., DECRISTOFORO, D. and UNGER, S. (1980) Detection and estimation of the degree of mitral regurgitation by pulsed Doppler echocardiography. *Circulation*, **61**, 143–147
12. KALMANSON, D., VEYRAT, C., ABITBOL, G. and FARJON, M. (1981) Doppler echocardiography and valvular regurgitation with special emphasis on mitral insufficiency. Advantages of two-dimensional echocardiography with real-time spectral analysis. In *Echocardiology*, edited by H. Rijsterborgh, pp. 279–290. The Hague: Martinus Nijhoff
13. TEIRSTEIN, P. S., YOCK, P. G. and POPP, R. L. (1985) The accuracy of Doppler ultrasound measurement of pressure gradients across irregular, dual, and tunnel-like obstructions to blood flow. *Circulation*, **72**, 577–584

6

Tricuspid valve disease

George Sutherland

Prior to birth the tricuspid valve lies between the low pressure right atrium and the systemic pressure right ventricle. Thus in the developing heart the tricuspid valve is, in effect, the systemic atrioventricular valve and must function in a way similar to the normal adult mitral valve (i.e. it must be both competent and non-stenotic). Morphologically the neonatal tricuspid valve appears poorly equipped for this function; in a term neonate it has a much larger orifice, very thin and comparatively poorly formed leaflets, and a subvalve tensor apparatus which appears rather tenuous when compared to the mitral subvalve apparatus.

Following birth and the rapid change from the fetal right heart dominated circulation to the dominant left heart circulation of the neonate, the haemodynamic role of the tricuspid valve changes dramatically. Within days of birth the pulmonary vascular resistance will fall to near normal levels resulting in a fall in right ventricular pressure in both systole and diastole. This fall in right heart pressure alters the flow velocities and flow profiles across the tricuspid valve. By about 3 months of age the right heart haemodynamics are stable and the right heart pressures and flow profiles remain basically unchanged during the remainder of normal life.

Congenital abnormalities of the tricuspid valve are relatively uncommon findings in paediatric cardiology; the application of prenatal cardiac scanning has demonstrated that most fetuses with severe tricuspid abnormalities are spontaneously aborted although a number do survive and are frequently born in severe cardiac failure. Congenital tricuspid stenosis as an isolated lesion is extremely rare. Stenosis and/or hypoplasia of the tricuspid valve in the neonate normally occurs as part of the spectrum of pulmonary atresia with intact ventricular septum and is most probably a consequence of the abnormal fetal flow patterns associated with that lesion. Congenital tricuspid regurgitation may be due to a primary abnormality of the tricuspid valve (such as Ebstein's anomaly) or to right ventricular dysfunction due to damage from either prenatal infection or intrapartum ischaemia, which frequently causes severe tricuspid regurgitation.

The most common form of tricuspid flow abnormality encountered in adult cardiology is secondary pathological tricuspid regurgitation. 'Physiological tricuspid regurgitation' is a normal finding in a high proportion of children and adults and is of no haemodynamic consequence, as discussed in Chapter 3 and later in this chapter. Pathological tricuspid regurgitation in the adult population, either of acute or chronic onset, is most commonly a result of significant left heart disease (either valvar, ischaemic or myopathic) or lung disease. Less frequently it is due to an intrinsic abnormality of the tricuspid valve itself, such as Ebstein's anomaly, tricuspid endocarditis or rheumatic tricuspid disease. Infrequently the latter may cause associated rheumatic tricuspid stenosis.

Evaluation of the nature of tricuspid valve disease and tricuspid haemodynamics prior to the introduction of Doppler was based on a combination of clinical examination, catheterization data and cross-sectional echocardiography. While the latter can provide reliable structural information in the diagnosis of lesions such as Ebstein's anomaly, tricuspid vegetations and rheumatic tricuspid stenosis, the images normally impart little in the way of accurate haemodynamic data. The diagnosis of tricuspid stenosis normally involves invasive dual catheter studies using high fidelity catheter tip manometers to give accurate pressure gradient evaluation. This is a technically difficult procedure, especially in patients with a stenotic tissue or mechanical tricuspid prosthesis. Similarly, both catheter pressure studies and angiographic data have proved unsatisfactory to differing degrees in the assessment of tricuspid regurgitation. Non-invasive assessment of the severity of both primary and secondary tricuspid regurgitation was considerably enhanced by the use of contrast echocardiography. Although a little cumbersome, and not strictly non-invasive, contrast echocardiography probably provided the most accurate assessment of the severity of tricuspid regurgitation prior to the introduction of duplex scanning[1, 2].

This chapter will attempt to assess the extent to which the introduction of Doppler has changed or revised our concept of tricuspid valve function and its investigation in both health and disease.

The examination of the normal tricuspid valve

Normal diastolic flow

Doppler signals from diastolic flow across the tricuspid valve are best recorded with the transducer in either an apical position or between the apex and the lower left sternal edge. The subcostal transducer position may not allow the transducer beam to be aligned to flow and it may be better to avoid it unless the precordial approach is unsatisfactory. Where duplex scanning is used it is normally a relatively straightforward matter to image the inlet of the heart in the four chamber view and identify the tricuspid valve. Using pulsed Doppler the tricuspid orifice can be scanned to achieve the best flow signals. Diastolic flow signals will be recorded immediately proximal to the tricuspid orifice in the floor of the right atrium; this represents atrial flow entering the tricuspid funnel. Scanning down between the tricuspid leaflets into the body of the right ventricle will demonstrate the valve clicks and slight acceleration in flow velocities as the sample volume is moved towards the ventricle. Appropriate use of the filter settings should give a clear tricuspid diastolic flow profile in virtually every patient studied.

Where non-imaging continuous wave Doppler is used, tricuspid flow is best recorded by placing the transducer in the apical position and identifying the characteristic mitral diastolic signal. The transducer can then be angled medially scanning on to the left ventricular outflow tract signal and then a medial and slightly posterior angulation of the transducer will normally record the characteristic tricuspid diastolic flow pattern. Non-imaging continuous wave Doppler can identify tricuspid diastolic flow in virtually every patient although duplex continuous wave Doppler certainly facilitates this examination for the inexperienced operator.

The normal tricuspid diastolic flow pattern is biphasic with the initial peak occurring immediately after tricuspid valve opening and the second peak occurring after atrial systole (*see* Chapter 3). In the preterm or term infant with persistence of the fetal vascular resistance or with parenchymal lung disease the second peak caused by atrial contraction is dominant and may achieve a peak velocity some two to three times the initial one. This is simply a result of the increased atrial contractility required to drive blood into the hypertrophied and non-compliant right ventricle. This dominance of atrial filling rapidly disappears with the reduction in right ventricular pressure (and hence increase in right ventricular compliance) as pulmonary vascular resistance falls. By one year of age the initial peak velocity is the higher of the two and this situation then holds true for the diastolic flow profile throughout the rest of normal life.

Another characteristic of normal tricuspid flow (and one which differentiates it from mitral flow) is the marked variation in both flow velocity and flow profile with normal respiration. Inspiration will increase tricuspid flow velocities throughout diastole and expiration will decrease them. It should be noted that maximal tricuspid diastolic velocity recorded in the normal heart will always be less than the maximal diastolic velocity recorded across the mitral valve, because the tricuspid orifice is invariably greater in size than the mitral orifice and mean flow across both is the same per cardiac cycle. Tricuspid peak velocity is normally some two-thirds of mitral peak velocity.

Physiological tricuspid regurgitation

Prior to the introduction of Doppler studies, both clinical examination and right ventricular angiography suggested that the normal tricuspid valve was not regurgitant. However, with the use of increasingly sophisticated spectral analysis, continuous wave Doppler has demonstrated the tricuspid valve to be 'physiologic-ally' regurgitant in between 35 and 46% of normal individuals studied. Therefore, it is necessary to consider what is meant by 'physiological tricuspid regurgitation'.

First, it should be stressed that this is a normal finding and does not indicate any intrinsic tricuspid valve dysfunction. Physiological tricuspid regurgitation is most easily recorded by continuous wave Doppler; the less sensitive pulsed Doppler mode fails to record the tricuspid waveforms in a significant number of patients where continuous wave succeeds[3]. The systolic waveform of physiological tricuspid regurgitation is most easily recorded using duplex continuous wave Doppler as the jet is remarkably constant in both the site of tricuspid origin and the direction of its extension into the right atrium. The inlet of the heart should be imaged and the tricuspid orifice, right atrium and atrial septum identified. The jet of physiological regurgitation will commence at the central point of systolic tricuspid leaflet coaptation and will be directed 1–3 cm posteriorly into the right atrium towards the lower third of the atrial septum. The jet extension or *jet length* can be confirmed by tracking it back using duplex pulsed Doppler or colour Doppler flow imaging (*see Plate 6*). The normal physiological tricuspid regurgitation waveform will be pansystolic with the peak velocity recorded between one-third and one-half way through systole (*Figure 6.1*). It is not always possible to demonstrate the complete velocity envelope with a clear cut maximal velocity which must be obtained prior to attempting to assess the pressure drop across the tricuspid valve (*see Figure 3.8*).

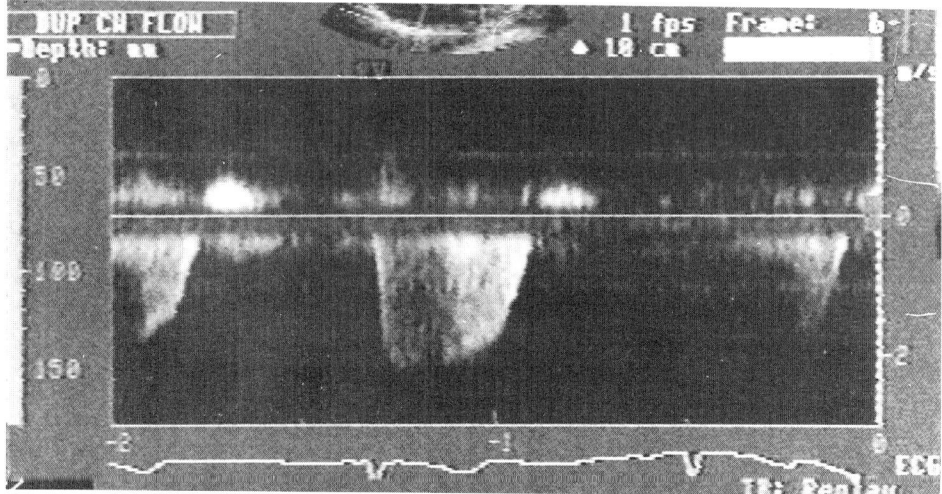

Figure 6.1 Signal of physiological tricuspid regurgitation from a patient with no significant heart disease

Physiological tricuspid regurgitation is difficult to record in preterm and newborn infants. This may be due, in part, to the high heart rate encountered in these patients but the low incidence (from personal experience <10% of patients studied) must be due to other factors. It may be that the neonatal tricuspid valve placed in a high pressure circuit has the same haemodynamic properties as the adult mitral valve in which physiological regurgitation is not recorded using precordial continuous wave Doppler. It appears that the incidence with which physiological tricuspid regurgitation can be recorded increases to a peak in adolescence but, thereafter, remains unchanged throughout normal life.

The maximal velocity of the tricuspid regurgitation jet can be used to estimate the peak systolic pressure in the right ventricle in every case where this is clearly recorded (*see* Chapter 3). The modified Bernoulli equation is applied to the maximum velocity to give the pressure drop from the right ventricle to atrium; if 5–10 mmHg are added to it for atrial pressure an estimate of the right ventricular pressure is reached[4]. In the absence of pulmonary stenosis this is equal to the pulmonary artery systolic pressure and is a useful means of assessing this. With normal right ventricular pressure (i.e. <30 mmHg) the peak velocity of the tricuspid regurgitation jet will be between 1.7 and 2.5 m/s. In clinical practice, it is frequently of great value in the assessment of cardiac or respiratory disease to record a normal tricuspid regurgitation peak velocity and thus be certain that the right heart pressures are normal.

Differentiation between pathological and physiological tricuspid regurgitation

When using Doppler it can be a problem to determine whether tricuspid regurgitation is physiological or mildly pathological. Less difficulty is encountered when distinguishing physiological from moderately severe tricuspid regurgitation. In a few cases it may be extremely difficult to determine the severity of pathological tricuspid regurgitation with sufficient accuracy to decide whether or not surgical intervention is required. However, although well-defined problem areas do exist,

Doppler may be used to assess the severity of tricuspid regurgitation with reasonable accuracy.

Several factors may be of value in assessing the severity of tricuspid regurgitation: (1) the peak systolic jet velocity; (2) the systolic velocity waveform; (3) the signal strength; (4) the extension of the tricuspid regurgitation jet into the right atrium, inferior vena cava and hepatic veins; (5) the jet width; (6) the appearance of the jet on colour flow mapping; (7) the diastolic tricuspid flow velocity and waveform.

If tricuspid regurgitation (either pathological or physiological) is present in an adolescent or adult, it should be possible to identify systolic backflow from right ventricle to right atrium in virtually every case when continuous wave Doppler is used. Where tricuspid regurgitation is physiological the peak velocity of the regurgitation jet will be less than 2.5 m/s (i.e. right ventricular peak systolic pressure will be normal). However, in up to 40% of cases where a tricuspid regurgitation signal is recorded, a complete velocity envelope may not be obtained and uncertainty may exist as to the precise peak systolic velocity. With an increase in tricuspid regurgitation from a mild to moderate degree the systolic waveform will remain the same, but the signal strength will normally increase. Where tricuspid regurgitation is physiological the regurgitation jet can be tracked back only some 2–3 cm into the right atrium using pulsed Doppler, the jet normally has no appreciable width, the jet never extends to the superior atrial wall, and no abnormal flow disturbance will be noted in the hepatic veins or inferior vena cava. When available, colour Doppler flow mapping can readily determine the origin, length and width of the physiological regurgitation jet and, thus, clearly distinguish this from significant pathological tricuspid regurgitation.

Pathological tricuspid regurgitation

Pathological tricuspid regurgitation may be due to a number of factors. It may occur as a result of organic tricuspid valve disease such as Ebstein's anomaly, rheumatic fever, or secondary to endocarditis. It is commonly found in patients with complete heart block. It is frequently present following right ventricular infarction in patients who may either have normal or elevated right heart pressure. Finally, tricuspid regurgitation may be due to either acute or chronic elevation of the right ventricular systolic pressure. In a study of over 400 patients with a broad spectrum of left heart disease the present author found the incidence of moderate to severe tricuspid regurgitation increased with the severity of the left heart disease, being present in 96% of those with severe ischaemic or valvar left heart disease, irrespective of the lesion. It must be emphasized that severe tricuspid regurgitation may occur both in the setting of a normal or an elevated right ventricular pressure with the latter being by far the more common finding.

Pathological, as opposed to physiological, regurgitation is normally associated with an increase in the intensity of the signal of the regurgitation jet, thus making it easier to record. However, this is not an invariable finding and, in cases where right atrial and right ventricular pressures are virtually equal (such as in the case of severe Ebstein's anomaly) and the cardiac output is low, the tricuspid regurgitation signal may be difficult to record despite the severity of the regurgitation. Pathological regurgitation is frequently associated with an elevation in the peak systolic jet velocity to values >2.6 m/s (indicating an elevated right ventricular systolic pressure). Where regurgitation is severe and there is early equalization of right ventricular and right atrial pressures there is a characteristic change in the regurgitation waveform (*Figure 6.2*) with a sharp rise to an early peak and a rapid fall in the velocity. This invariably indicates severe tricuspid regurgitation. When right ventricular dysfunction is the direct cause of the pathological regurgitation the initial rate of rise in the velocity waveform may be reduced (*Figure 6.3*) when

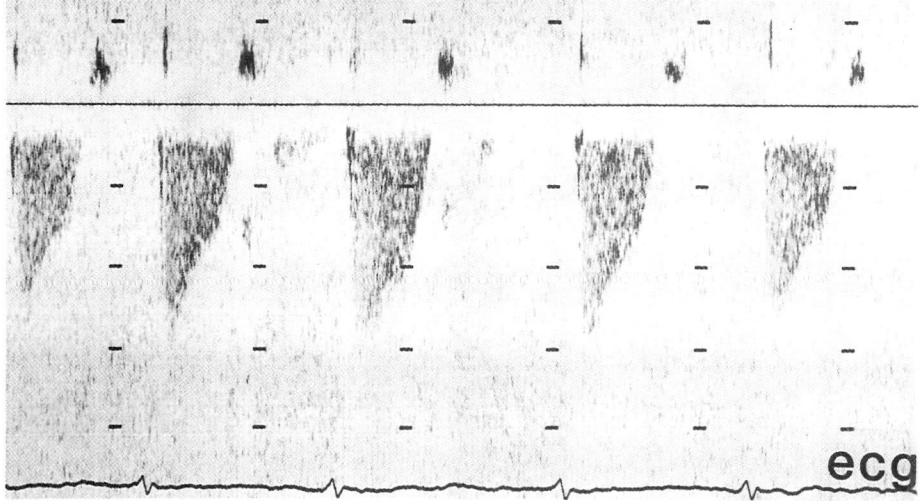

Figure 6.2 Continuous wave Doppler in severe tricuspid regurgitation. The waveform shows a sharp initial rise with a very early fall off due to the rapid equalization of right atrial and ventricular pressures. The respiratory variation in the peak systolic velocity (average 2.8 m/s) is clearly apparent

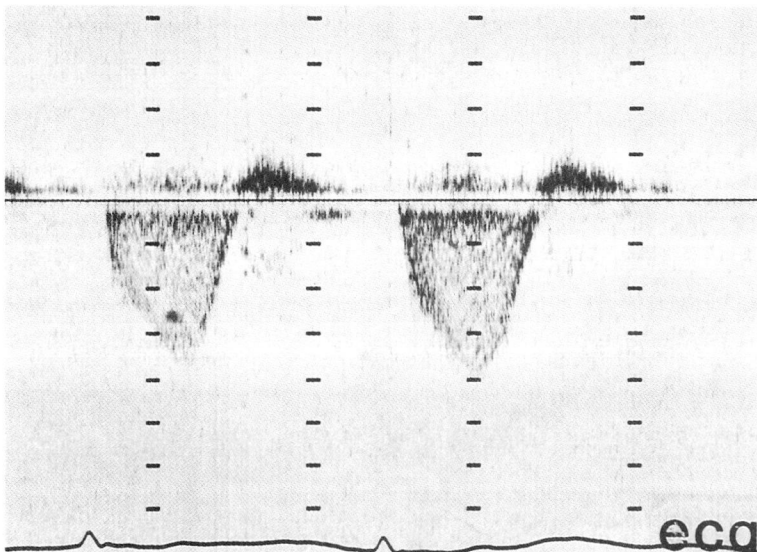

Figure 6.3 Continuous wave Doppler waveforms in moderate tricuspid regurgitation. The systolic waveform shows a complete velocity envelope allowing the right ventricular pressure to be estimated. Peak velocity = 3.7 m/s, calculated right ventricular peak systolic pressure = approximately 50 mmHg

compared with the patient with normal ventricular function. The regurgitation waveform may be similarly altered by the presence of ventricular premature beats (*Figure 6.4*). Although peak velocity, systolic waveform and signal strength are of value in assessing the severity and cause of the tricuspid regurgitation, all may be misleading. More information can often be derived from both the jet length and width within the right atrium, and the jet extension into the inferior vena cava and

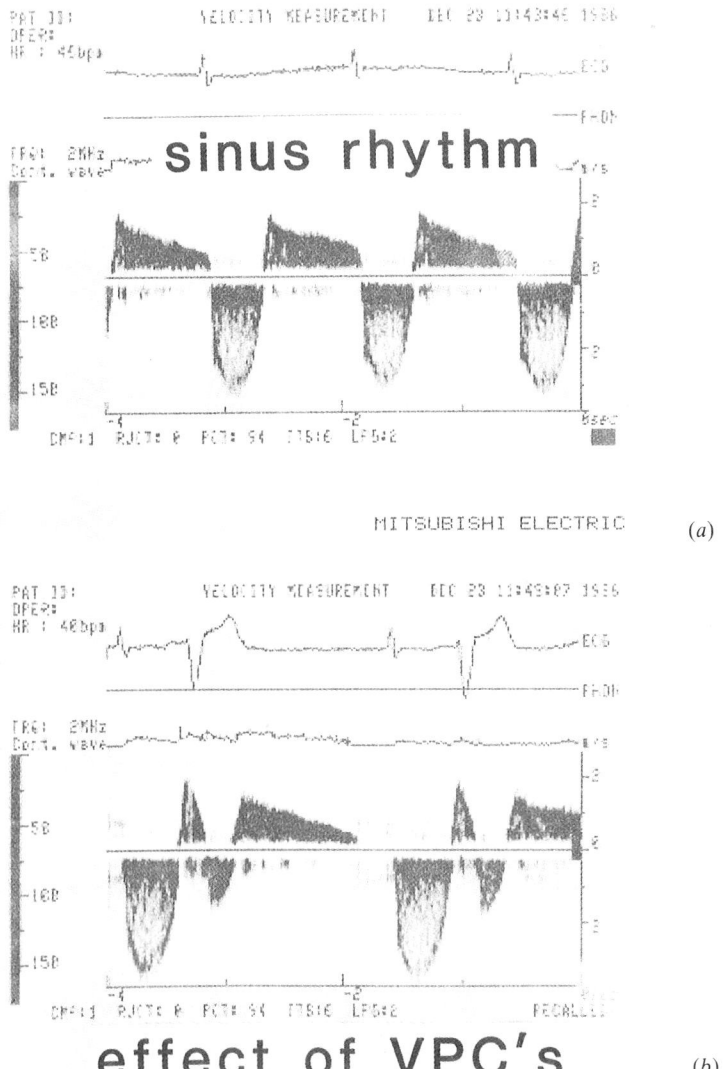

Figure 6.4 Continuous wave waveforms in a patient with tricuspid stenosis and regurgitation. (*a*) With the patient in sinus rhythm the prolonged pressure half-time characteristic of tricuspid stenosis is demonstrated and the regurgitation waveform is typical of moderate tricuspid regurgitation with a peak velocity of 3.1 m/s. (*b*) With ventricular premature contractions (VPCs) the postectopic beat shows the apparent reduction in the pressure half-time and fall in the end diastolic gradient. In addition, in the ectopic beat there is a fall in the velocity of the tricuspid regurgitation jet and change in the waveform with a rapid reduction in velocity indicating severe tricuspid regurgitation

hepatic veins. A tricuspid regurgitation jet tracked back to the superior atrial wall or into the hepatic veins using pulsed Doppler invariably indicates severe tricuspid regurgitation[1, 2, 5]. Colour Doppler flow mapping has greatly simplified this evaluation, showing both the extent and width of the regurgitant jet (*see Plate 7*) and its extension down into the hepatic veins (*see Plate 8*).

Abnormal tricuspid diastolic flow velocities and waveforms

The peak velocity of flow across the tricuspid valve may be increased to abnormal values where the valve is hypoplastic, stenotic or prosthetic, or the valve is normal and there is either increased flow across it or the right ventricle is non-compliant.

Increased flow across a structurally normal valve is best exemplified by the pandiastolic velocity increase associated with the left to right shunt of a secundum atrial septal defect (*see* Chapter 8). Although this increases velocity throughout diastole the major effect is to increase the early diastolic velocity with the peak in some cases reaching 2.3 m/s. The calculated pressure half-time is not altered. High flow situations tend to eliminate the respiratory variation in the tricuspid waveform which occurs with normal flow. The finding of an increased tricuspid early diastolic velocity greater than that of the mitral valve at the corresponding point in diastole

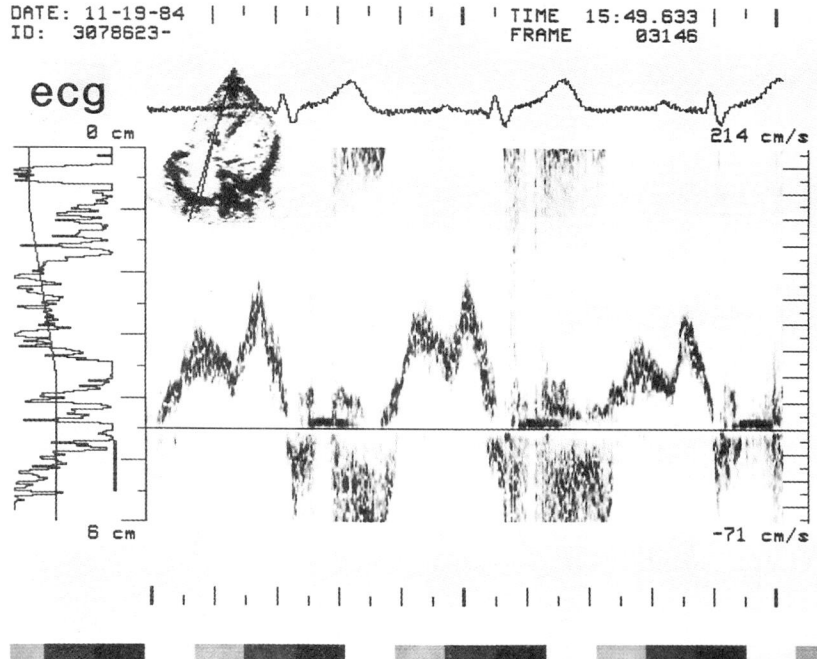

Figure 6.5 Pulsed Doppler recording of the tricuspid valve flow pattern in a patient with pulmonary atresia and intact ventricular septum. Atrial contraction produces a late diastolic peak in the tricuspid diastolic flow as a result of the very non-compliant right ventricle. Systolic aliasing, which indicates high velocity tricuspid regurgitation, is present

is strong evidence of a significant atrial shunt in patients with a secundum atrial septal defect or partial anomalous pulmonary venous drainage.

The tricuspid peak velocity may be abnormally increased in late diastole in patients with a non-compliant right ventricle or severe tricuspid stenosis (a very rare lesion). This late diastolic velocity increase is due to atrial contraction and is only present in patients who are in sinus rhythm. It is frequently encountered in children with severe lung disease, severe pulmonary vascular disease or with severe right ventricular outflow tract obstruction (*Figure 6.5*). It is less commonly found in adult patients.

Tricuspid hypoplasia is an extremely rare lesion. The flow abnormalities are similar to those encountered in patients with increased flow across a structurally normal valve. The pressure half-time has been within normal limits in all three patients with this lesion whom the present author has studied.

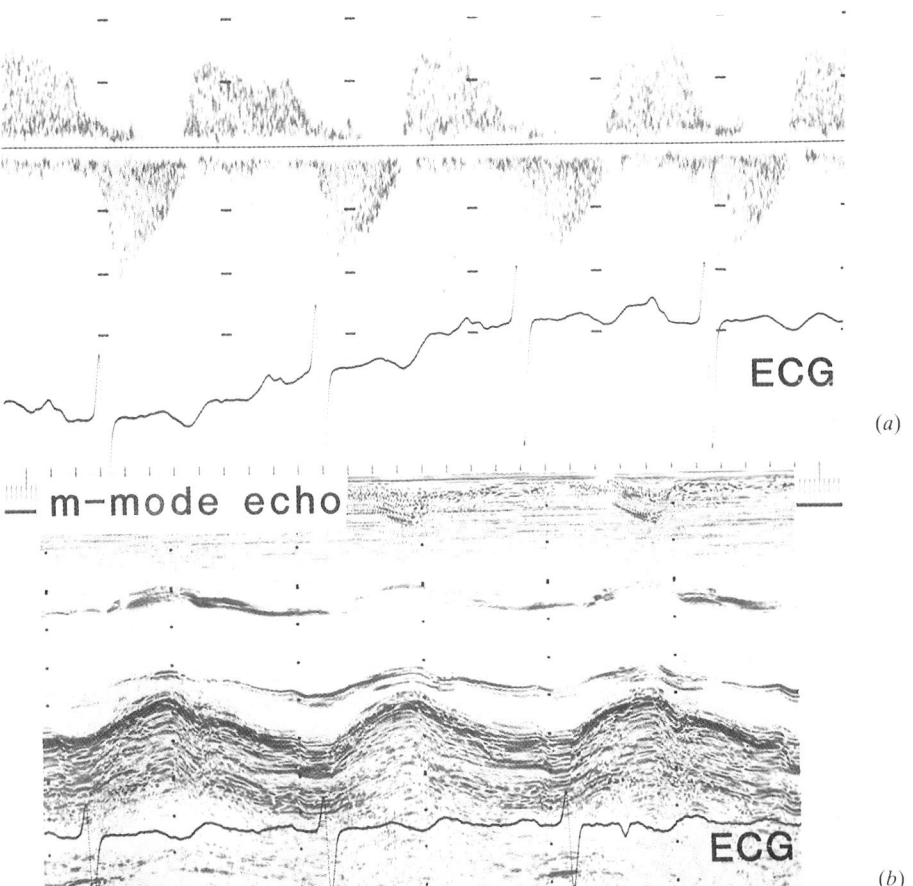

Figure 6.6 Studies from a patient with carcinoid syndrome with moderate tricuspid stenosis and severe regurgitation. (*a*) Early and rapid fall in systolic velocity of severe tricuspid regurgitation and slow fall in diastolic velocity with prolonged half-time of stenosis. (*b*) M-mode echocardiogram of the dilated right ventricle and tricuspid valve. The tricuspid valve leaflets are widely separated with their rigidity holding the valve widely open during the whole cardiac cycle

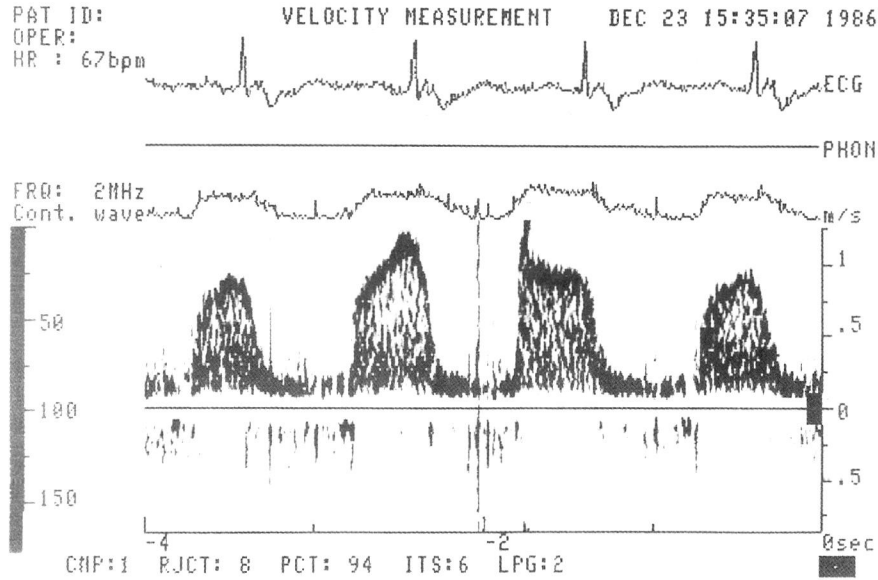

Figure 6.7 Grossly abnormal waveforms from a tricuspid heterograft. In addition to tricuspid stenosis, there is gross right ventricular dysfunction with severe elevation of the right ventricular end diastolic pressure. The combination of both of these results in marked changes in the diastolic waveforms during the respiratory cycle

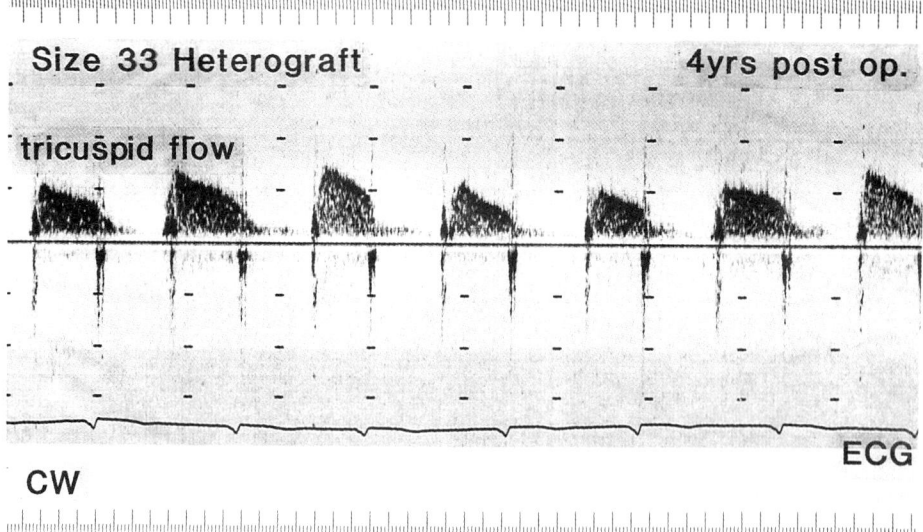

Figure 6.8 Continuous wave Doppler recording from a tricuspid heterograft from a patient in sinus rhythm. Mild tricuspid prosthesis stenosis is present with moderate prolongation of the pressure half-time. The waveform is characteristic for the prosthesis. No tricuspid regurgitation was recorded in this case. Note that the typical respiratory variation in the velocity waveform is retained

Tricuspid stenosis

Doppler is probably the most sensitive technique available to the cardiologist with which to diagnose tricuspid stenosis. Imaging remains unreliable in many cases and frequently even dual high fidelity manometer tip catheter studies are misleading. Continuous wave and pulsed Doppler are equally effective in ascertaining the diagnosis; the tricuspid velocities are higher than normal with persistence of a pressure gradient throughout diastole. There is usually a slow decrease in velocity during diastole and the pressure half-time is significantly prolonged (*Figures 6.4, 6.6 and 6.7*). The calculated mean pressure drop is derived in the same manner as for the mitral valve (*see* Chapter 5), but for the tricuspid valve lower values for the mean pressure drop (i.e. >3 mmHg) can be taken to represent severe obstruction. An increase in the mean pressure drop is normally very noticeable during inspiration with a corresponding fall with expiration. It is probably best to estimate the mean pressure drop and pressure half-time in the middle of the respiratory cycle, taking the average of five such beats. Tricuspid regurgitation may increase the mean pressure drop in patients with tricuspid valve disease but, as with mitral stenosis, neither the velocity waveform nor the pressure half-time will suggest tricuspid stenosis.

Tricuspid valve prostheses

All tricuspid prostheses, either mechanical or bioprosthetic, are mildly stenotic[6] (*see* Chapter 9). Each will have its own flow characteristics including velocity profile, normal mean pressure drop and pressure half-time (*Figure 6.8*). Since large series of findings in normal tricuspid prostheses are not yet available, these should be recorded in each case following operation and prosthetic function can then be monitored at appropriate intervals. The appearances in prosthetic tricuspid stenosis are similar to those in native valves and the criteria for assessing the severity are similar.

References

1. LIEPPE, W., BEHAR, V. S., SCALLION, R. and KISSLO, J. A. (1978) Detection of tricuspid regurgitation with two-dimensional echocardiography and peripheral vein injections. *Circulation*, **57**, 128–132
2. MELTZER, R. S., VAN HOOGENHUYZE, D., SERRUYS, P. W., HAALEBOS, M. M. P., HUGHENHOLTZ, P. G. and ROELANDT, J. (1981) Diagnosis of tricuspid regurgitation by contrast echocardiology. *Circulation*, **63**, 1093–1099
3. BENCHIMOL, A., HARRIS, C. L. and DESSER, K. B. (1973) Non-invasive diagnosis of tricuspid insufficiency utilizing the external Doppler flowmeter probe. *Am. J. Cardiol.*, **32**, 868–873
4. CURRIE, P. J., SEWARD, J. B., CHAN, K. L. *et al.* (1985) Continuous wave Doppler determination of right ventricular pressure: a simultaneous Doppler-catheterisation study in 127 patients. *J. Am. Coll. Cardiol.*, **6**, 750–756
5. VEYRAT, C., KALMANSON, D., FARJON, J., MANIN, J. P. and ABITBOL, G. (1982) Noninvasive diagnosis and assessment of tricuspid regurgitation and stenosis using one and two dimensional echo-pulsed Doppler. *Br. Heart J.*, **47**, 596–605
6. HAERTEN, K., SEIPEL, L., LOOGEN, F. and HERZER, J. (1978) Haemodynamic studies after De Vega's tricuspid annuloplasty. *Circulation*, **58** (Suppl. 1), I28–I33

7

Pulmonary valve disease

Alan B. Houston

Abnormalities of the right ventricular outflow tract are nearly always the result of developmental anomalies and thus tend to present early in life. Most frequently the clinical problem is due to an obstructive lesion at valve or subvalve level, but obstruction can occur more distally with some congenital abnormalities or following pulmonary artery banding. Pulmonary regurgitation is uncommon as a primary or isolated problem, but it is becoming more important as a sequel to surgery, particularly repair of tetralogy of Fallot with a transannular patch.

In addition to its value in assessing pulmonary valve lesions, Doppler recording of the signal of pulmonary valve regurgitation, even in patients without pulmonary valve disease, can be of practical use in the assessment of pulmonary artery pressure since measurement of the peak velocity of the regurgitant jet allows calculation of the diastolic pressure difference across the valve.

Thus Doppler interrogation of the right ventricular outflow tract may be of value in the assessment of pulmonary stenosis, pulmonary regurgitation and pulmonary artery pressure.

Pulmonary stenosis

Pulmonary stenosis as an isolated abnormality accounts for about 10% of the total of congenital heart defects and is a relatively frequent association with a variety of other abnormalities, both cyanotic and acyanotic. When pulmonary stenosis occurs as an isolated lesion patients are asymptomatic unless the obstruction is severe. With significant stenosis the murmur is loud and a routine medical examination usually suggests congenital heart disease before or soon after school entry. Thus, in the developed countries, the management of pulmonary stenosis is largely the responsibility of the paediatric cardiologist but, occasionally, the condition may not be recognized until later in life and, in addition, the care of those who have undergone treatment of pulmonary stenosis in childhood will increasingly become the remit of the adult cardiologist.

Clinical examination should establish the diagnosis, but is of limited use in determining its severity. Moderate to severe pulmonary stenosis is suggested by a loud murmur, a soft second sound and a right ventricular heave or hypertrophy on an electrocardiogram (ECG). It is less easy to determine the severity of mild to moderate obstruction when there is only an ejection systolic murmur and the ECG is often normal. Attempts to estimate pressure gradient by measurement of the interval from the Q wave of the ECG or the first heart sound to an ejection click, or the width of splitting of the second heart sound are relatively insensitive. Similarly echocardiography is of little value; the depth of the A wave of the pulmonary valve on M-mode is of no practical value, and the presence of doming of the pulmonary valve and post-stenotic dilatation on two-dimensional echocardiography simply confirms the basic diagnosis.

Doppler with its unique ability to measure transvalvar gradients now provides an easy, accurate and reproducible means of assessing the severity of pulmonary stenosis.

Technique

A two-dimensional echocardiogram should first be obtained to confirm the diagnosis and, by demonstrating the intracardiac anatomy, suggest positions from which the Doppler beam might most accurately be aligned along the right ventricular outflow. This position can be utilized initially, but since pulmonary flow can be obtained from a variety of positions, the maximum velocity can only be obtained with certainty by exploring all possible sites and not just using the mid or upper left sternal edge from which a good short axis two-dimensional image or M-mode pulmonary valve recording can be made. The maximum velocity signal may be obtained as flow away from the transducer from the second left interspace downwards or from a subxiphoid position. Very occasionally it is best shown as flow towards the transducer in the first left interspace, the subclavicular area, or suprasternal notch. In some of these positions considerable tilting of the transducer is required to obtain the flow signal and a stand alone transducer is likely to be easier to manipulate than one within the head of a duplex system. This occurs particularly from the subcostal position where the transducer may have to be tilted in such a way that only part of its face is in contact with the skin or ultrasound jelly.

With moderate to severe pulmonary stenosis the high flow velocity signal exceeds the Nyquist limit and is best obtained with a continuous wave (CW) transducer; imaging may be of little help and may even cause confusion in deciding the position from which the best signal can be obtained. It can be easier to start with continuous wave to obtain the maximum velocity signal and use imaging with simultaneous pulsed or high pulsed repetition frequency (PRF) Doppler to localize the increased velocity to just beyond the valve ring.

Figure 7.1 is a typical recording in pulmonary valve stenosis obtained with continuous wave Doppler from a subxiphoid position from a child with pulmonary valve stenosis, a lower velocity having been obtained from parasternal positions. The maximum velocity of 4.8 m/s (equivalent to a gradient of 92 mmHg) is too high to be recorded by the pulsed technique but high PRF showed it to originate just at the valve. With continuous wave alone a similar flow signal will be obtained from those with a pulmonary artery band, or fixed subvalve or supravalve obstruction.

Right ventricular outflow tract (RVOT) obstruction is not always discrete but may occur at multiple levels, most frequently found with tetralogy of Fallot when there can be associated subvalve, valve and supravalve obstruction. With continuous wave Doppler a signal similar to that obtained with discrete stenosis is usually obtained, allowing the total gradient to be estimated with the simple modified Bernoulli equation but giving no information about the severity at

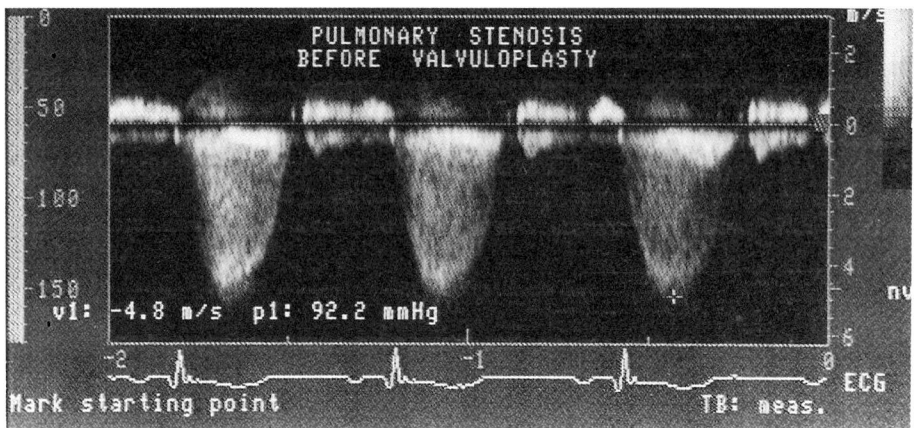

Figure 7.1 Spectral recording obtained from a subxiphoid position from a child with pulmonary valve stenosis. The maximum velocity of 4.8 m/s corresponds to a gradient of 92 mmHg

different levels. Tracking with pulsed Doppler can demonstrate an increased velocity at the level of the initial obstruction and a further increase distally, but this is a difficult procedure for obtaining accurate information. Colour Doppler is likely to be particularly valuable in demonstrating the position at which the high velocity occurs and thus the site of obstruction.

In infants and young children pulmonary infundibular stenosis may be dynamic rather than fixed, increasing throughout systole. This does not usually occur on its own but with infundibular muscular hypertrophy in response to a more distal obstruction. Under these circumstances Doppler ultrasound shows a different wave form, exhibiting a slower rise and an upstroke concave rather than convex. With distal fixed obstruction minor adjustments of the transducer, often tilting slightly medially, will produce a signal similar to that with fixed obstruction which will give the total right ventricle to pulmonary artery pressure drop with the slower rising infundibular signal superimposed upon it (*Figures 7.2* and *7.3*).

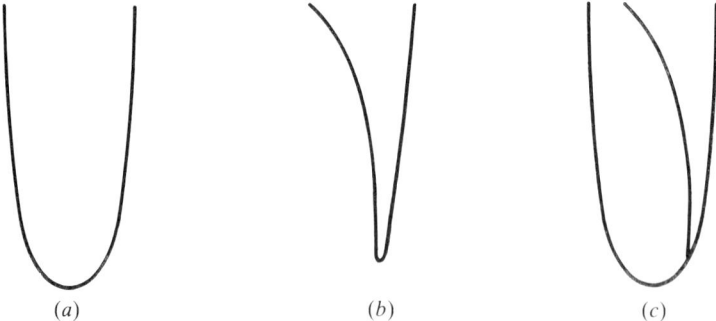

(*a*)   (*b*)   (*c*)

Figure 7.2 Diagrammatic representation of the wave forms in fixed and dynamic obstruction. With fixed obstruction, whether at valve level or above or below, the signal has a convex up and down stroke (*a*). With dynamic obstruction the upstroke is concave (*b*) but by adjusting the transducer position it is usually possible to obtain a spectral signal with the two waveforms superimposed (*c*)

Pulmonary regurgitation

Congenital pulmonary regurgitation is uncommon, generally only occurring with idiopathic dilatation of the pulmonary artery or absence of the pulmonary valve, usually with a ventricular septal defect (VSD). Acquired pulmonary regurgitation is a much more frequent finding as the result of pulmonary valvotomy or outflow reconstruction for tetralogy of Fallot. With severe regurgitation there may be cardiomegaly or a right ventricular heave, but these signs are non-specific and of limited discriminative value. Echocardiography has an important role in assessing the severity; pulmonary regurgitation causes right ventricular dilatation and the M-mode study will show right ventricular volume overload, manifest as paradoxical septal motion with the degree of right ventricular dilatation giving an estimate of the regurgitant volume.

Pulmonary regurgitation (which cannot be recognized clinically) can be recorded in about 10% of normal subjects (see Chapter 3) and, although of little clinical significance, is found in about 50% of patients with a variety of pulmonary and left heart lesions which cause pulmonary hypertension. In this situation, assessment of the severity of pulmonary regurgitation is of little importance but Doppler can be used to provide a non-invasive assessment of pulmonary artery diastolic pressure.

Technique

The signal of pulmonary regurgitation is usually obtained from a similar position to that used to record pulmonary systolic flow. It is easily obtained with moderate or severe regurgitation but when this is mild, as in normal subjects or secondary to pulmonary hypertension, the spectral signal can be less easy to record. This is one situation where stand alone continuous wave Doppler may be less sensitive than imaging with pulsed Doppler; the regurgitant flow is generally recorded just proximal to the valve near the inferior edge of the outflow tract. Clear recognition of the regurgitation is readily obtained with colour Doppler flow mapping which is particularly useful in demonstrating the position and direction of the jet (see Plate 9) thus permitting spectral studies to be performed. Pulmonary regurgitation has its highest velocity early in diastole and then falls progressively, sometimes with an extra dip following atrial contraction (see Chapter 3, Figures 3.9 and 3.10). In some, the full spectral signal cannot be obtained and only the earliest part of the signal is apparent.

Assessment of the severity of regurgitation through the pulmonary valve is fraught with all the difficulties that apply to other sites and accurate quantitation of the flow volume is not possible. In general, as with other situations, the more severe the regurgitation the more easily will the signal be picked up, the greater its intensity (Figure 7.4), and the further its extension into the right ventricle. With severe regurgitation the velocity falls to almost zero in end diastole as the pressures in the pulmonary artery and the right ventricle become equal (Figure 7.4). In addition, with pulsed or colour Doppler, retrograde diastolic flow will be demonstrated extending more distally into the pulmonary artery and its branches (see Plate 10).

With pulmonary hypertension a similar signal occurs but it is of higher velocity, maximal in early diastole and falls relatively slowly until end diastole (Figure 7.5). By applying the Bernoulli equation to this velocity throughout diastole, an estimate of the pressure difference between the pulmonary artery and right ventricle during this period is obtained. Since the right ventricular pressure in diastole is very low this approximates to the pulmonary artery diastolic pressure.

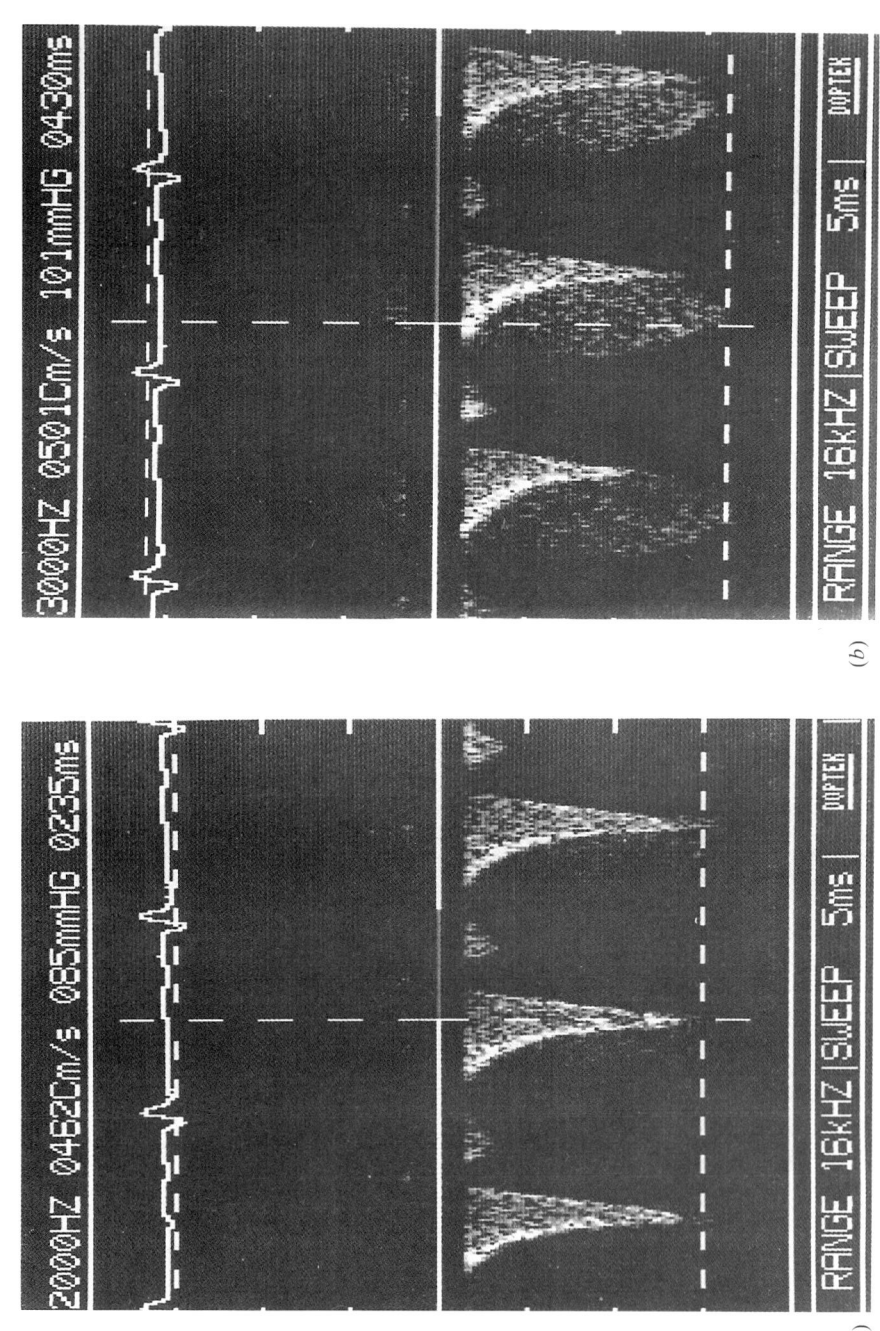

(b)

(a)

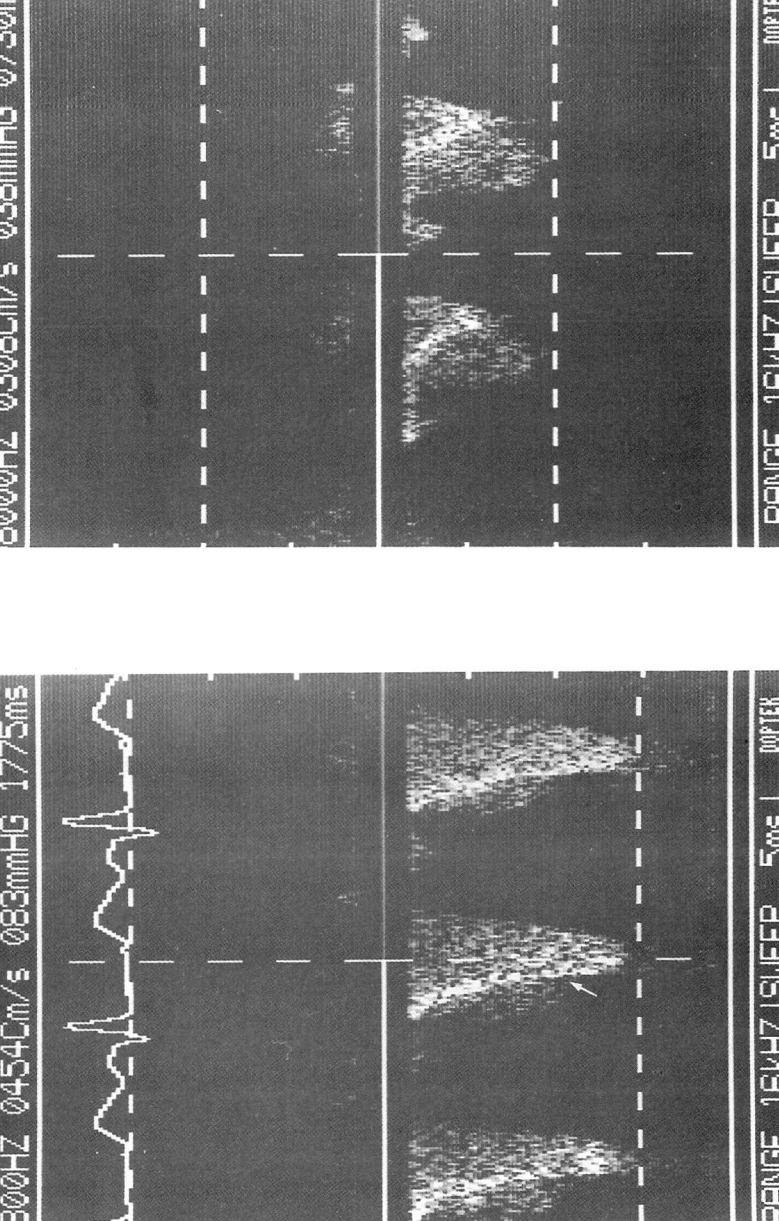

Figure 7.3 Spectral recording from a 3-month-old child with severe pulmonary valve stenosis in whom angiocardiography demonstrated severe pulmonary valve stenosis with marked infundibular dynamic obstruction. Before valvuloplasty the typical concave signal of dynamic obstruction (*a*) is apparent and minor change in angulation shows this superimposed on the signal of fixed obstruction (*b*). Immediately after valvuloplasty and 2 days later the total gradient is still high (*c*) but mainly due to dynamic obstruction, the fixed component of 3.3 m/s (arrow) suggesting a good result from the valvuloplasty. The good result is confirmed 6 weeks later (*d*) when the fixed gradient is equal to 38 mmHg with the dynamic gradient having regressed to only 16 mmHg

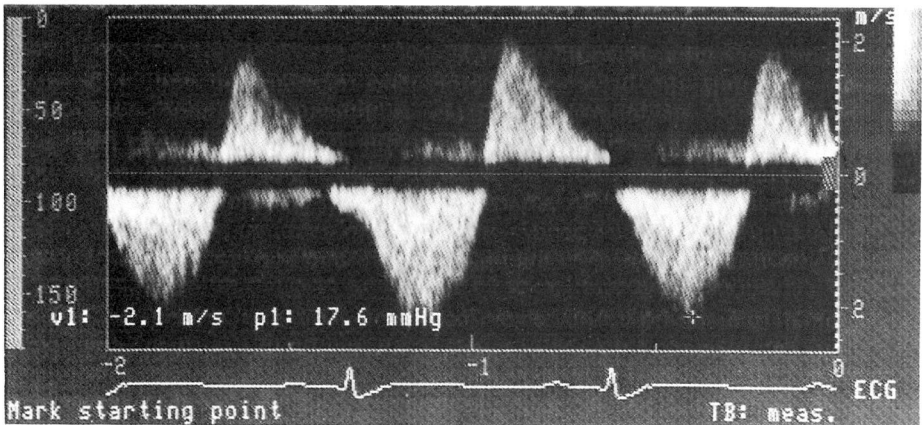

Figure 7.4 Signal of pulmonary regurgitation from a child of 6 years with severe pulmonary regurgitation following pulmonary valvotomy as a neonate for pulmonary atresia with intact ventricular septum. The maximum velocity is normal indicating normal pulmonary artery diastolic pressure. Significant regurgitation is suggested by the high intensity and rapid fall to almost zero in end diastole

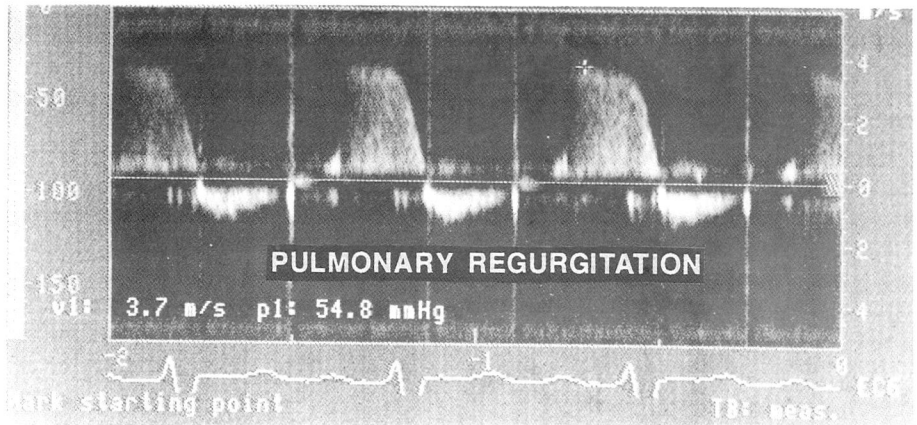

Figure 7.5 Recording of pulmonary regurgitation from a man with systemic level pulmonary hypertension. The full diastolic signal is not recorded but there is a maximum velocity of at least 3.7 m/s indicating a high pulmonary artery diastolic pressure

Clinical applications

Good Doppler signals of pulmonary flow can virtually always be obtained from children and young adults, the subcostal position being particularly useful if lung interference causes difficulties in parasternal positions. In adults, satisfactory Doppler studies may be recorded even when good M-mode records of the pulmonary valve cannot be obtained; when there is difficulty, asking the patient to lie in a lateral position with breath held in expiration may be useful.

Several reported studies of patients with discrete obstruction have confirmed a good correlation with gradient measured at catheterization[1–3]; this is excellent when pressure is measured simultaneously with two catheters, one on each side of the pulmonary valve[4], emphasizing the accuracy of Doppler. Doppler may show a minor degree of overestimation and minor discrepancies can occur with non-simultaneous records, particularly those performed at different times with different degrees of sedation. Possible overestimation of gradient related to the difference between peak-to-peak and instantaneous maximum velocities, although important in aortic stenosis (*see* Chapter 4), is of little significance in pulmonary stenosis since the relatively low pulmonary artery pressure throughout systole results in only a small difference. For practical clinical purposes this can be ignored and it is appropriate to consider Doppler as being virtually equivalent to the conventionally measured peak-to-peak pressure in those with pulmonary stenosis. It should always be remembered that in the presence of right ventricular volume overload (which can be demonstrated by echocardiography), the subvalve velocity must be considered in calculating the gradient or it may be overestimated.

In applying this technique to clinical practice it must be considered that although surgical treatment of pulmonary valve stenosis has been considered necessary if the gradient across the valve is greater than 40–50 mmHg, the introduction of valvuloplasty may change these criteria, making the treatment of those with lesser gradients dependent on the practice in an individual unit. Doppler estimate is so accurate that catheterization is not now necessary to distinguish patients with mild or unimportant pulmonary stenosis from those in whom the obstruction is at a level requiring relief by valvuloplasty or surgery. If the Doppler gradient is greater than 50 mmHg the obstruction will require relief, while if it is less than 30 mmHg it will be of little importance. A value of between 30 and 50 mmHg would suggest that the obstruction is not severe and it might therefore be appropriate to consider valvuloplasty or to perform serial Doppler examinations and defer possible treatment until a later date.

The measurement is equally accurate in calculating the pressure across a pulmonary artery band. Doppler is of particular value in the follow-up of patients who have undergone this procedure in whom initial clinical improvement can be slow, raising the question of the efficacy of the band.

The problem of the patient with RVOT obstruction at multiple levels is of interest to the paediatric cardiologist dealing with infants and young children but, since they usually undergo surgery early, it is of little relevance to those dealing with older children and adults. In most of these patients clinical and echocardiographic assessment indicate the need for angiocardiography or surgical treatment but there are others in whom the degree of infundibular stenosis changes with time and a non-invasive technique for performing serial measurement of the obstruction will be important.

In cases with obstruction at multiple levels, Doppler and measured gradients have proved less comparable[5] than in those with discrete obstruction. This seems to be due to problems of pressure measurement and probably does not indicate any inherent problem with the application of the Bernoulli formula in this situation; *in vitro* studies seem to have confirmed this[6]. Doppler ultrasound cannot yet determine the relative importance of the valve or fixed subvalve stenosis, but the decision on the need for surgical treatment is based on the total gradient and, to the surgeon, knowledge (echocardiographic or angiocardiographic) of the right ventricular outflow tract and pulmonary artery anatomy is much more necessary than physiological information on the relative contributions of the infundibulum and valve to the total obstruction.

Persons who are unfamiliar with the principles of the Bernoulli formula have shown surprise that it provides accurate values in patients such as those with tetralogy of Fallot where, with time, there can be considerable variation in the severity of the infundibular stenosis with major changes in the volume of blood flowing through the right ventricular outflow. However, in these patients, the pulmonary artery pressure is low and relatively constant and the right ventricular pressure, which is at systemic level, will show only relatively small changes and thus the pressure gradient will change little. The Bernoulli formula measures the pressure drop which is related to the increase in velocity and is independent of size of orifice (unless it is very small) and therefore provides an accurate prediction of the gradient.

A cardiologist or physician in the more developed parts of the world will only rarely be referred an adult patient presenting for the first time with significant pulmonary stenosis, but may see some with a murmur due to mild or moderate obstruction or, increasingly in the future, those who have undergone pulmonary valve surgery earlier in life. In the former group, Doppler should be applied in a similar way to that previously discussed and providing that satisfactory signals are obtained a good estimate of the obstruction will be obtained.

Follow-up after treatment

This group of patients is likely to include both those who had a valvotomy or valvuloplasty for valve stenosis and those who required a RVOT patch for more severe obstruction such as tetralogy of Fallot. Right bundle branch block is common and the ECG is of little value in assessing right ventricular hypertrophy. They may have not only mild residual pulmonary stenosis, but also pulmonary regurgitation which can often present more of a clinical problem. The Bernoulli equation will estimate the gradient and, although marked regurgitation may result in increased forward flow in systole with possible overestimation if the proximal velocity is not considered, it will not fail to recognize anyone with significant residual obstruction. Pulmonary regurgitation can be demonstrated by Doppler but, although quantitation into mild, moderate, or severe is theoretically possible, it is difficult to provide a more detailed assessment. The echocardiographic display of an enlarged right ventricle with paradoxical septal motion indicating right ventricular volume overload is perhaps more useful in demonstrating it is of significant degree and following its progress. However, the decision as to who requires a pulmonary valve replacement can be difficult and ultrasound does not give the definitive answer.

Doppler may be of particular value in assessing the result of valvuloplasty, particularly where there is a secondary dynamic infundibular obstruction. Following valvuloplasty the gradient may not fall to its final value immediately and Doppler allows serial assessment to be performed and indicates the relative contribution of the fixed and dynamic obstruction. *Figure 7.3* illustrates this in a 3-month-old infant before and after valvuloplasty. Outpatient study suggested a total gradient of 120 mmHg and when sedated for catheterization this was 100 mmHg (5 m/s) with a concave signal indicating a dynamic element to this equivalent to 85 mmHg (4.6 m/s). One hour after valvuloplasty the Doppler signal still attained a maximum velocity of 4.77 m/s (equivalent to 91 mmHg) with the upstroke still showing a concave pattern but wider character. Two days later the dynamic obstructive signal had a maximum of 4.5 m/s but angulation of the transducer more medially showed a superimposition of a fixed obstructive signal of only 3.2 m/s; this implies that the valve obstruction has been well dealt with (fixed gradient approximately 40 mmHg), but there is still significant infundibular hypertrophy with a dynamic gradient of about 80 mmHg which is almost the same as previously. Six weeks later the infundibular signal had virtually disappeared (2 m/s) and there remained a fixed one (3.1 m/s) equivalent to 38 mmHg which would have been predicted from Doppler from the waveform 2 days after valvuloplasty. In most cases the changes are much less dramatic than this but when they do occur Doppler allows a simple and accurate assessment.

Although it seems likely that the pulmonary diastolic pressure can be estimated with Doppler there is as yet no detailed study confirming this and it is perhaps better for the meantime simply to examine the tracing and note the high velocity rather than translate this into an absolute pulmonary artery diastolic pressure as would be measured at catheterization.

Thus Doppler is a reliable means of determining the severity of pulmonary stenosis and precludes the need for catheterization to obtain a gradient measurement. It is a very sensitive means of demonstrating pulmonary regurgitation but adds little to present techniques in determining its severity. On occasions it may be helpful in giving an estimate of the pulmonary artery diastolic pressure but this is often apparent from other investigations and is of limited clinical value.

References

1. LIMA, C. O., SAHN, D.J., VALDES-CRUZ, L. M. *et al*. (1983) Non-invasive prediction of transvalvular pressure gradient in patients with pulmonary stenosis by quantitative two-dimensional echocardiographic Doppler studies. *Circulation,* **67,** 866–871
2. JOHNSON, G. L., KWAN, O. L., HANDSHOE, S., NOONAN, J. A. and DE MARIA, A. N. (1984) Accuracy of combined two-dimensional echocardiography and continuous wave Doppler recordings in the estimation of pressure gradient in right ventricular outlet obstruction. *J. Am. Coll. Cardiol.,* **3,** 1013–1018
3. HOUSTON, A. B., SHELDON, C. S., SIMPSON, I. A., DOIG, W. B. and COLEMAN, E.N. (1985) The severity of pulmonary valve or artery obstruction in children estimated by Doppler ultrasound. *Eur. Heart J.,* **6,** 786–790
4. CURRIE, P. J., HAGLER, D. J., SEWARD, J. B. *et al*. (1986) Instantaneous pressure gradient: a simultaneous Doppler and dual catheter correlative study. *J. Am. Coll. Cardiol.,* **7,** 800–806
5. HOUSTON, A. B., SIMPSON, I. A., SHELDON, C. D., DOIG, W. B. and COLEMAN, E. N. (1986) Doppler ultrasound in the estimation of the severity of pulmonary infundibular stenosis in infants and children. *Br. Heart J.,* **55,** 381–385
6. TEIRSTEIN, P. S., YOCK, P. G. and POPP, A. L. (1985) The accuracy of Doppler ultrasound measurement of pressure gradients across irregular, dual and tunnel-like obstructions to blood flow. *Circulation,* **72,** 577–584

8

Congenital heart disease

Alan B. Houston

The management of congenital heart disease is to a large extent the province of the specialist paediatric cardiologist. The most severe and complex abnormalities present in the first weeks or months of life, often undergo investigation and surgery in infancy or early childhood, and do not present diagnostic problems to the general physician or cardiologist. However, the presence of less severe forms of congenital heart disease may not be recognized until school age or even adult life. Patients can then be seen by a cardiologist without specialist experience in paediatric cardiology, a general physician or paediatrician who may refer them directly to the physiological measurement department of a general hospital for non-invasive assessment, in particular ultrasound studies. This chapter is designed to be of help to the general reader rather than the specialist paediatric cardiologist and considers mainly the more common acyanotic lesions which may not be referred directly to the paediatric cardiologist.

Accurate assessment of congenital heart disease requires both a clear demonstration of the intracardiac and great artery anatomy and accurate knowledge of the physiological effects of the lesion. In the complex, often cyanotic, lesions anatomical information is usually of paramount importance and echocardiographic demonstration of the lesion is usually sufficient to allow the majority of sick infants to undergo surgery without catheterization. However, in other lesions, usually acyanotic, and in older children surgical decisions are more often dependent on physiological information such as transvalvar gradient, pulmonary artery pressure, and shunt size. Echocardiography cannot provide this information, but Doppler has the potential ability to do so.

For diagnostic purposes the common forms of acyanotic congenital heart disease can be subdivided into those with a left to right shunt (ventricular septal defect (VSD), patent ductus arteriosus (PDA) and atrial septal defect (ASD)), and those with an obstructive lesion (pulmonary and aortic stenosis and coarctation of the aorta). This chapter considers the application of Doppler ultrasound to these defects and, for the non-specialist, gives a very brief description of presentation, clinical findings and problems for each lesion.

In most lesions Doppler is applied in one or more of three ways: the calculation of the pressure gradient from the modified Bernoulli formula; the provision of information additional to that of the echocardiogram on the site of the lesion; the quantitation of shunt size. The basic principles of shunt measurement apply to all lesions with an intracardiac shunt and, to a large extent, are determined by the measurement of ventricular output (*see* Chapter 10). This aspect is worth considering briefly rather than discussing it independently for each individual defect.

Estimation of pulmonary to systemic flow ratio

The calculation of the pulmonary to systemic flow ratio (QP/QS) from oximetry and the Fick principle has been one of the main objectives of the invasive assessment of congenital heart disease with left to right shunts. However, when comparing Doppler-derived measurement with that obtained at catheterization it must be remembered that the catheterization value is in itself subject to error and is not necessarily an exact measurement, particularly in the atrial septal defect where the mixed venous oxygen is impossible to measure accurately.

The principles and problems in the measurement of volumetric flow are discussed in detail in relation to cardiac output in Chapter 10. They apply to the measurement of both pulmonary and systemic flow and thus the calculation of QP/QS. The mean flow velocity is determined with pulsed Doppler, usually with the sample volume at the valve ring, and the area is measured from echocardiography. Since satisfactory images of the lateral wall of the pulmonary artery may not be obtained, it is sometimes not possible to measure its area (and thus flow) directly, but pulmonary flow can then theoretically be gauged by examining another valve which has the same volumetric flow (i.e. the tricuspid in ASD or mitral in VSD). Furthermore, when the intracardiac shunt occurs at different levels, the pulmonary and systemic flow have to be measured from different sites. In ductus arteriosus aortic flow equals mitral flow which is total pulmonary blood flow and not systemic flow. Thus systemic flow can be measured in VSD as aortic or tricuspid flow, in ASD as mitral or aortic flow, and in PDA as tricuspid or pulmonary flow, while pulmonary flow is measured in VSD as mitral or pulmonary flow, in ASD as tricuspid or pulmonary flow, and in PDA as mitral or aortic flow. Assessment of atrioventricular valve flow is difficult because the valve areas cannot be measured accurately, so where possible, shunt calculation should be made using values obtained from the ventricular outlets.

Published results have shown satisfactory correlation with measured ratios in most lesions[1], but these come from studies generally performed by an operator dedicated to spending time to obtain a perfect study and, of course, those who do not obtain such good results are less likely to publish this. There are inherent difficulties in the measurement of both velocity and area and, in addition to the inaccuracies discussed in the measurement of cardiac output, there is twice the chance of an error since the measurement is made at two sites. The results will be less reproducible by different technicians and physicans than other Doppler measurements such as maximum velocity. The problems in the application of this are such that it is important that, where possible, each department attempts to validate the technique and the physician is wary of the significance to put on a Doppler measurement of QP/QS, unless the accuracy of the technique in the reporting department has been validated. Indeed, some may consider that the technique is more of a research tool and, although it can be helpful in some selected cases, in practical terms Doppler measurement of QP/QS adds little to the non-invasive evaluation of congenital heart disease. As with all aspects of Doppler, the technique should not be considered in isolation and a reasonable estimate of shunt size, sufficient for clinical purposes, may often be obtained from clinical or echocardiographic examination.

Aortic and pulmonary stenosis

The use of Doppler in outlet valve stenosis has been discussed in detail in Chapters 4 and 7. In children, the technique is generally more easily applied than in adults and good quality records can be obtained from most subjects from a variety of sites.

In isolated pulmonary valve stenosis, the Doppler estimate of gradient should be very accurate and clinical decisions can be based on this result alone. Doppler can also be valuable when pulmonary stenosis occurs as part of a more complex lesion, particularly when it is not possible to, or considered inappropriate to attempt to, enter the pulmonary artery.

In aortic stenosis the same reservations on the comparison of Doppler and catheterization measurements apply to children and adults, and the Doppler value should not be considered to be equivalent to a peak-to-peak measurement at catheterization. However, because of the ease of obtaining signals from a number of sites there is less chance of Doppler underestimating the instantaneous gradient in aortic valve stenosis. As yet there is no confirmation of the accuracy in a large series of patients with subaortic stenosis and the author's experience has suggested that Doppler may underestimate the true instantaneous gradient in this situation, possibly because of the unusual angle or short extension of the jet through the subaortic obstruction.

Ventricular septal defect

The ventricular septal defect is the most common congenital cardiac lesion, accounting for over one-quarter of the total number of defects. The management of patients with a VSD presents two distinct problems; in the young child the decision to be made is if and when closure should be undertaken, and in the older child with a small VSD that the defect is present and prophylaxis against infective endocarditis is required.

In the majority of cases the clinical diagnosis of VSD is not difficult, but echocardiography is necessary to rule out associated abnormalities and provide a detailed anatomical diagnosis, demonstrating the site and size of moderate or large lesions[2]. Surgical closure is clearly indicated at any time in infancy if the VSD causes intractable cardiac failure or failure to thrive, and is also considered necessary before the age of 2 years when the pulmonary vascular resistance is increased. Thus the decision as to whether surgical closure is necessary is dependent on physiological information, the pulmonary artery pressure and shunt size. A large shunt is suggested by clinical or radiological cardiomegaly, an apical mid-diastolic murmur and left ventricular hypertrophy on ECG or enlargement on echocardiography. Pulmonary hypertension is likely when there is a right ventricular heave and loud second sound and ECG evidence of right ventricular hypertrophy. With M-mode echocardiography measurement of right-sided systolic time intervals, in particular pre-ejection period divided by ejection time, is of some help. However, although all these techniques, including clinical examination, clearly demonstrate the extremes, there is considerable overlap in the intermediate cases and precise determination of the pulmonary artery pressure requires catheterization and its direct measurement.

Doppler ultrasound with its ability to measure volumetric flow and pressure differences can be applied in several ways to the assessment of the patient with a

VSD; it can provide an estimate of both the pulmonary pressure and shunt size and, by showing flow through the septum, can confirm the presence of defects not apparent on imaging.

Technique

With Doppler the demonstration of the presence of a VSD and the most useful means of assessing pulmonary artery pressure requires that flow through the septum is recorded. This can be performed with either pulsed[3] or continuous wave[4] Doppler. Although a two-dimensional echocardiogram will demonstrate the septum and, in most patients, the position of a significant VSD, it must be remembered that, as in other conditions, it only gives a guide to the optimal position and angulation for recording maximum velocity of flow. The entire left parasternal edge and the subxiphoid position must be explored and the position and angulation of the probe adjusted to obtain the maximum velocity signal. Even when using an imaging system with steerable continuous wave Doppler it is often easier to use continuous wave alone to explore for the flow signal.

When the optimal signal has been found, pulsed or high pulsed repetition frequency (PRF) Doppler can then be used to give an optimal record and imaging to demonstrate the exact site of origin of the flow signal. With pulsed Doppler it is important to track the flow disturbance through the septum since a similar finding can occur on occasions on either side of the septum in the absence of a VSD[3]. The signal is often best obtained from a low left parasternal or subxiphoid position and continuous wave Doppler shows that the maximum velocity occurs in mid-systole, falls to almost zero just after aortic closure and continues usually with low velocity flow through diastole (*Figure 8.1*). There can be an early to mid-diastolic increase in flow velocity which, with continuous wave Doppler, may sometimes be due to

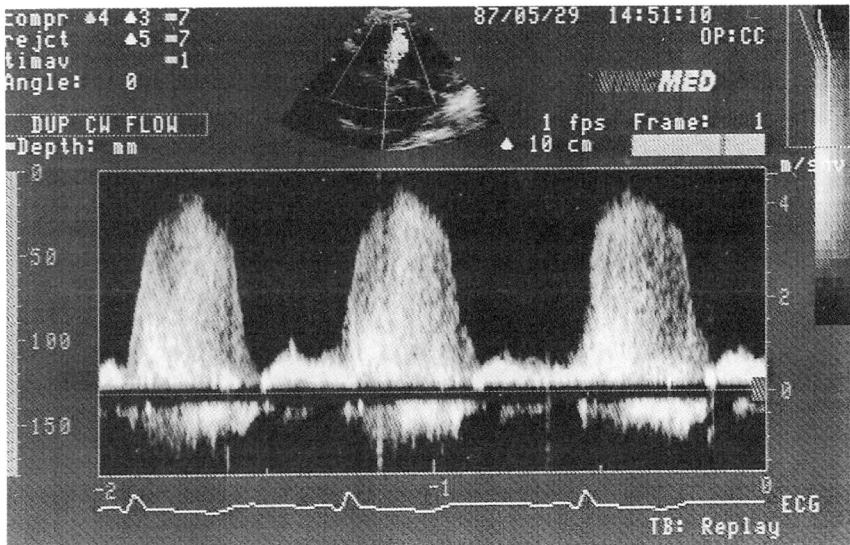

Figure 8.1 Continuous wave recording from a patient with a small membranous ventricular septal defect. The maximum velocity of 4.3 m/s which occurs in systole is equivalent to a pressure difference of 74 mmHg indicating a low pulmonary artery pressure

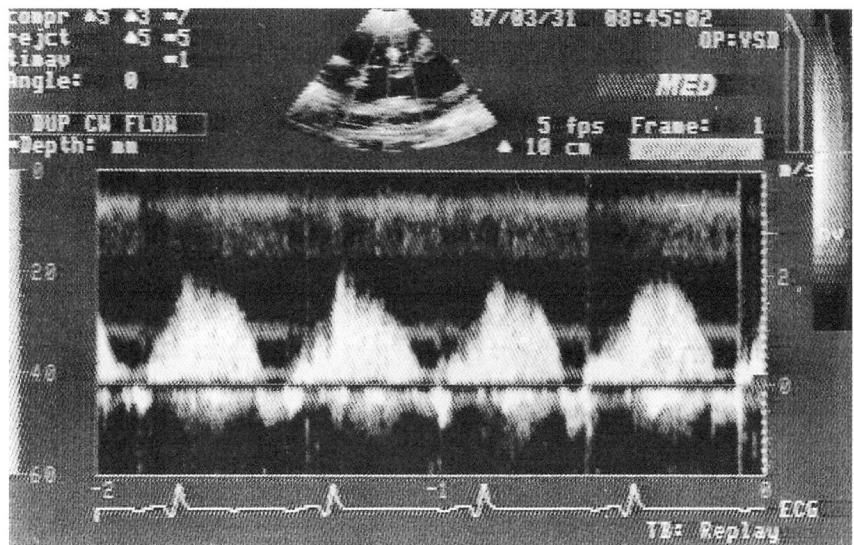

Figure 8.2 Continuous wave recording from an infant with a large ventricular septal defect, high flow and pulmonary hypertension. Flow occurs throughout the cardiac cycle with a maximum velocity of approximately 2 m/s indicating that there is little pressure difference (16 mmHg from the Bernoulli equation) between the ventricles and that there is pulmonary hypertension at almost systemic level

the superimposition of mitral valve flow. If the pressure difference between the ventricles is small the signal is of low velocity but, providing there is a left to right shunt, it will still be possible to demonstrate it (*Figure 8.2*). In the vast majority of cases the signal is positive indicating flow towards the transducer but, on occasions, particularly with muscular defects, the jet emerges from the septum at such an angle that it is directed away from the transducer. When there is a high velocity jet it is not always possible to obtain a complete spectral envelope with a single transducer angulation but slight alteration of its position should show both the upstroke and downstroke, though not necessarily simultaneously, and permit the maximum velocity to be measured. Occasionally with small muscular defects a complete spectral signal is not obtained and the maximum velocity cannot then be measured. In patients with a VSD, adjustment of the machine settings can be important and, in particular, the high pass filter may need to be set to its maximum to exclude high amplitude, low velocity signals which can often swamp the lower amplitude, high velocity ones in a VSD.

The estimation of pulmonary artery pressure is then based on the premise that the systemic blood pressure equals the left ventricular systolic pressure and Doppler can measure the interventricular gradient[4, 5]; subtraction of this from the systolic blood pressure will give the right ventricular, and in the absence of pulmonary stenosis, the pulmonary arterial systolic pressure. Comparison of the pressure drop from the left to right ventricle estimated by the Bernoulli equation and measured at catheterization shows a relatively good correlation, but this is not as close as in outlet valve stenosis. Where the pressure drop is greater than 50 mmHg, an underestimation can be obtained in more than half, this usually but not always being less than 20 mmHg (*Figure 8.3*); these patients have small defects and the direction of the jet varies with cardiac contraction such that the Doppler

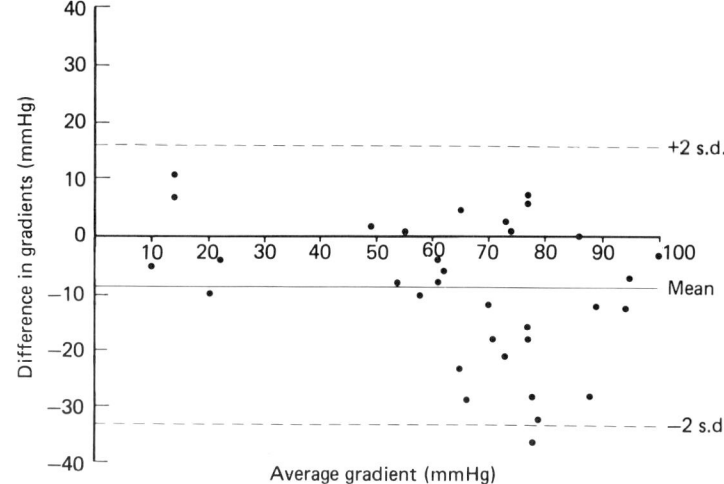

Figure 8.3 Comparison of the difference between the Doppler and instantaneous gradients with the average of the gradients in patients with a ventricular septal defect

beam cannot always be optimally aligned with it. Should the instantaneous gradient be significantly greater than the peak-to-peak, Doppler would be expected to overestimate the pressure drop; however, simultaneous ventricular pressure measurements have shown little variation between these and it is of little clinical significance and, for practical purposes, it seems appropriate simply to consider the Doppler estimate as being similar to the peak-to-peak.

Although the pulsed and continuous techniques when used with imaging can demonstrate VSD position it can be difficult to identify more than one defect. Colour Doppler will show the VSD site more precisely (*see Plates 11, 12 and 13*) and should also allow more than one jet to be picked up with greater certainty[6], although it is not infallible.

After demonstrating and measuring the velocity of VSD flow, study of the patient with a VSD should include assessment of pulmonary and tricuspid flow. Measurement of systolic velocity at pulmonary valve level is necessary to exclude stenosis; as always when the velocity at valve level is increased it must be measured in the subvalve area to ensure the increase is not simply the result of increased flow due to the shunt. The recording of pulmonary regurgitation when possible will give an estimate of pulmonary artery diastolic pressure (*see* Chapter 7). Tricuspid regurgitation can be difficult to record in patients with a VSD but should be sought as a further means of assessing right ventricular and thus pulmonary arterial pressure (*see* Chapter 6).

The pulmonary/systemic flow ratio can be calculated from the respective ventricular outputs. A number of reported studies testify to the value of the technique, but it is subject to all the potential errors of output measurement (*see* Chapter 10) and since this applies to each different site the potential for error is considerable. In addition, the presence of turbulent flow in the pulmonary artery as the result of the VSD can further complicate this investigation and pulmonary flow may have to be measured at the mitral valve where area measurement is fraught with problems.

Clinical application

The most useful application of Doppler in patients with a VSD is in the assessment of pulmonary arterial pressure to allow selection of those likely to require surgical closure. However, since patients falling into this group are almost invariably under the age of 2 years, their management is the responsibility of the paediatric cardiologist and of little concern to the general physician or cardiologist. However, a VSD can develop in older patients following a myocardial infarction or penetrating chest injury.

The pulmonary artery pressure can be assessed with Doppler by the measurement of interventricular pressure drop or right-sided valve regurgitation. In those with a VSD, the most straightforward and repeatable method and thus most likely to be accepted in routine practice, is by subtraction of the ventricular gradient from the systemic blood pressure to obtain the right ventricular and pulmonary arterial pressure and this does indeed give a reasonable assessment. There is a tendency for Doppler to underestimate high pressure differences but, since this will give a false high right-sided pressure, cases of pulmonary hypertension should not be missed. Of major clinical importance should be overestimation of the drop with subsequent underestimation of right ventricular pressure; there is no good evidence for this in patients with high right ventricular pressures. Thus Doppler does appear to provide more information than other non-invasive methods, but it is prudent to consider that for the meantime reliance on Doppler alone is inappropriate. Each laboratory still needs to consider its own expertise and results and, as yet, should consider Doppler only as one part of the total non-invasive study in these infants.

The major drawback to this technique is the measurement of blood pressure in the infant or toddler; poor cooperation may make this extremely time consuming if not impossible. Sedation may be necessary thus detracting from its value as a routine outpatient investigation. However, continuous wave Doppler will usually pick up a reasonable VSD signal and a clinical assessment can be based on this value. If it is accepted that most patients under 2 years old have a systolic blood pressure less than 110 mmHg (95th centile) and that those with a right ventricular pressure less than 50% of the left will not require surgery, a Doppler record of 55 mmHg or below should not miss any child with pulmonary pressure at a level requiring operation, while one less than 30 mmHg is likely to be associated with a ventricular pressure drop below 30 mmHg and thus high pulmonary pressure. As with other techniques the difficult group is those with a Doppler record between 30 and 55 mmHg and Doppler has not yet been shown to be sufficiently accurate to allow a distinction between those who will or will not require surgery. Blood pressure measurement may be necessary and of course factors such as flow volume, which allow pulmonary vascular resistance to be calculated, need to be considered, particularly in the intermediate group. If tricuspid regurgitation can be recorded and the pressure estimate from this agrees with that from the former technique this is strong evidence that the assessment is likely to be accurate.

In the older asymptomatic patient with a murmur, clinical examination often gives conclusive evidence of a VSD but, in others, it can be difficult to decide whether the murmur is innocent or due to a small VSD. In virtually all patients with a normal right ventricular pressure careful Doppler study will pick up the jet, even in those in whom the defect is not apparent on echocardiography. Indeed Doppler is so sensitive that a VSD flow signal can occasionally be demonstrated in patients with a small defect in whom no murmur is audible. Thus the detection of a Doppler signal of a VSD is an extremely (if not the most) sensitive technique for detecting flow through, and thus demonstrating the presence of, a small VSD. This may allow a more rational approach to the management of the asymptomatic patient, preclude the unnecessary use of antibiotic prophylaxis and permit early discharge from follow-up. In this respect colour Doppler may well prove to be more valuable than continuous wave alone and indeed it is likely that they will be complementary.

Patent ductus arteriosus

The ductus arteriosus which accounts for about 12% of acyanotic congenital heart disease tends to cause symptoms only in the first 6 months of life, occasionally producing cardiac failure or failure to thrive in infancy, or contributing to the ventilatory requirements of the preterm infant with respiratory problems.

Beyond the neonatal period the diagnosis is usually easily made by the presence of the typical murmur but it may be difficult to detect this when there is another loud murmur (e.g. a VSD), or the murmur may be atypical in some circumstances such as the presence of pulmonary hypertension which, by altering the usual pressure difference between the great arteries, modifies the murmur and makes it soft, short or atypical. With a significant shunt a chest X-ray will show non-specific increase in pulmonary vascularity and cardiomegaly; an indentation on the left side of the trachea would be more specific evidence for the diagnosis. The electrocardiogram (ECG) can show non-specific changes; left ventricular hypertrophy is consistent with a significant shunt at ventricular or great artery level and right ventricular hypertrophy with pulmonary hypertension. M-mode echocardiography can demonstrate increased left atrial and ventricular size and the two-dimensional image may demonstrate the ductus arteriosus, although this is not always possible.

Doppler ultrasound is likely to be of confirmatory value in most patients but it may be of diagnostic value in some where the diagnosis of ductus arteriosus is uncertain and, in addition, it may assist in establishing the pulmonary pressure.

Technique

With imaging and pulsed Doppler a short axis view of the great arteries can be used and the sample volume placed in the distal main pulmonary artery where normal systolic flow away from the transducer through the pulmonary valve occurs, but diastolic flow towards the transducer suggests ductal flow[7]. However, the maximum velocity flow signal may be obtained from a higher position, the first or second left interspace or suprasternal notch where imaging can be difficult. It is usually obtained with continuous wave Doppler and can be picked up without difficulty using a stand alone transducer[8]. With low pulmonary artery pressure this signal characteristically shows continuous flow with maximum velocity in systole falling to a lower velocity in diastole (*Figure 8.4*). The auditory signal is remarkably similar to a ductus arteriosus on auscultation with a stethoscope. The velocity of this signal reflects the pressure difference between the great arteries. The diastolic velocity is usually relatively high but occasionally may be low, in the range of 1 m/s, similar to that of coarctation.

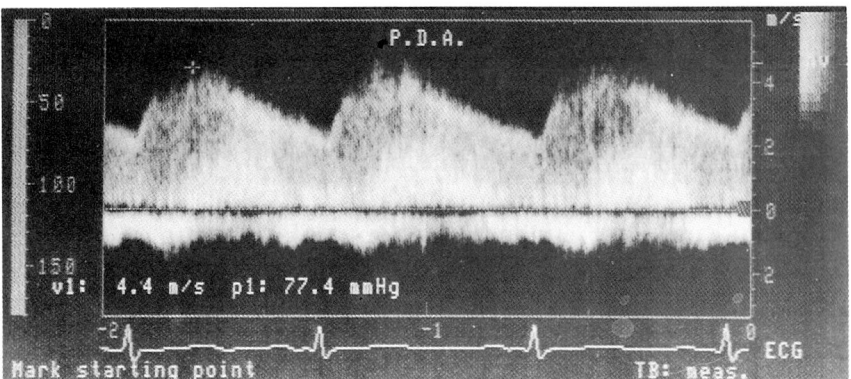

Figure 8.4 Continuous wave Doppler recording from a high parasternal position from a patient with a patent ductus arteriosus (PDA). The beam is aligned along the duct and shows continuous flow throughout the cardiac cycle

Occasionally, when there is pulmonary hypertension the pressure difference between the great arteries can be altered, being greater in diastole, with the result that the Doppler signal has a higher velocity in diastole than systole. Under these circumstances imaging and pulsed Doppler is helpful but the diagnosis is more certain if colour Doppler is used to demonstrate flow through the ductus arteriosus and align the beam directly in the direction of flow (*see Plate 14*).

If the pulsed wave sample volume is positioned in the descending aorta or neck vessels, reversed flow in diastole should be apparent where there is significant diastolic flow through the ductus. However, under these circumstances continuous wave Doppler will more clearly demonstrate ductal flow and, indeed, a high pulse pressure will be apparent on clinical examination. Thus this has little practical application.

The ductus arteriosus flow signal is usually easily picked up, but it must be remembered that a similar wave form can be obtained from approximately the same site in other conditions in which there is continuous flow; this will be away from the transducer in coarctation of the aorta or left pulmonary artery stenosis (both of which will have a relatively low diastolic velocity which is only rarely found with a ductus), but towards it in flow through an aortopulmonary window, a collateral artery in coarctation, a major aortopulmonary collateral artery in pulmonary atresia or a Blalock–Taussig shunt. Careful use of imaging and high PRF (or colour) Doppler should resolve any such difficulty and since these lesions (apart from the aortopulmonary window) have different clinical signs any confusion as to the source of the signal should not arise. If Doppler has difficulty distinguishing a patent ductus arteriosus from aortopulmonary window contrast echocardiography should resolve the diagnosis. In some conditions, such as pulmonary atresia, flow through the ductus tends to be at a different angle, away from and not towards the transducer when it is positioned in the suprasternal notch.

The velocity of the flow signal can be used to estimate both the systolic and diastolic pressures in the pulmonary artery by applying the Bernoulli equation to calculate the gradient between the great arteries and subtracting this from the blood pressure measured with a sphygmomanometer. However, this has not proved as accurate as in the VSD, presumably because of difficulties in obtaining the optimum angulation.

Clinical application

In the common situation of the child with the classical signs of ductus arteriosus including a continuous murmur, chest X-ray, ECG and echocardiography in keeping with the diagnosis, surgery can easily be recommended without catheterization even if the ductus is not clearly demonstrated by echocardiography. Here Doppler adds little to the clinical assessment and decision making. However, it is another useful adjunct and it could be argued that Doppler demonstration of a clear duct signal (which will also allow estimation of pulmonary pressure) is more useful than an ECG or chest X-ray, providing echocardiography excludes other abnormalities.

Experience with Doppler has, however, proved it to be much more sensitive than clinical examination or other non-invasive means in detecting the presence of a ductus arteriosus and it can demonstrate very small lesions where experienced cardiologists who know the diagnosis cannot detect the murmur. In this situation it might be suggested that ligation is not necessary, but perhaps it is illogical to leave these lesions but still recommend closure on the grounds of possible infective endocarditis in small ducts with low flow and no pulmonary hypertension where a murmur is audible.

When there is pulmonary hypertension with low velocity flow the signal can be less easy to record and the use of an imaging transducer is almost essential. There is as yet not enough evidence dogmatically to state the sensitivity of Doppler in this situation, but it is likely that, providing there is flow through the duct, conventional (and probably colour Doppler) will provide significant information which is additional to that already available non-invasively on the presence of a ductus arteriosus in this situation.

With the preterm infant the use of Doppler suffers from the same problem as echocardiography with difficulty obtaining signals from the suprasternal notch and upper left sternal edge as the infant is undergoing intensive care on a ventilator and hyperinflated lungs interfere with signal transmission. In these infants, the therapeutic question is not the presence of a patent ductus but its significance in terms of pulmonary flow and clinical effects. Although Doppler may demonstrate ductal flow, attempts to quantitate it and measure QP/QS can be particularly fraught with inaccuracies in these tiny babies and as yet firm recommendations cannot be given.

The ductal flow signal has different characteristics when it occurs in association with other lesions and this can be useful in their assessment. Thus with pulmonary atresia it generally has the same waveform, but can appear as flow away from the transducer from the suprasternal notch and even the left sternal edge. Where the flow is through the ductus from pulmonary artery to aorta, as in severe coarctation (or pulmonary hypertension), flow will mainly be the reverse of normal, and indeed may be misinterpreted as through the coarctation. However, even in the situation of aortic atresia where all systemic flow is from the pulmonary artery via the PDA to the aorta there tends to be some diastolic backflow from the aorta to the pulmonary artery.

An assessment of shunt size can be obtained by determining pulmonary flow from the mitral and aortic valves (i.e. the pulmonary venous return) and systemic flow from the tricuspid or pulmonary valves (i.e. the systemic venous return). However, an idea of this can be obtained from the size of the left-sided chambers and the measurement of pulmonary artery pressure or pulmonary/systemic flow ratio is less important in ductus arteriosus since it is generally considered appropriate that these cases are all ligated even if the defects are small with low flow and normal pulmonary pressure. Where there is doubt about the pulmonary pressure it seems that the Doppler estimation of the maximum systolic pressure drop between the great arteries from the maximum velocity signal should not be relied upon for calculating the pressure.

Atrial septal defect

The atrial septal defect, which comprises 10% of all forms of congenital heart disease, is perhaps the most difficult lesion to recognize with clinical examination. Patients are usually asymptomatic until at least the second decade and clinical signs such as the wide fixed splitting of the second sound, the ejection systolic murmur in the pulmonary area and the tricuspid mid-diastolic murmur are often most unimpressive. Since the murmur can be very soft, patients with an ASD may be considered to have an innocent murmur or not even recognized to have one, and thus the presence of heart disease may not be recognized until well into later life. The chest X-ray may show increased vascularity but does not always show a characteristic appearance. In most cases with an ostium secundum defect an rsR' complex is shown on the ECG and, although this is not universally found, if there is the slightest suspicion of an ASD, its presence is a strong indication for performing an echocardiogram. The introduction of echocardiography has transformed the diagnosis of atrial septal defect and some paediatric cardiologists who practised before echocardiography may have had reason to wonder whether they dismissed a number of patients with an ASD as having an innocent murmur.

If there is a significant left to right shunt at atrial level the M-mode echocardiogram will show an increased right ventricle dimension with paradoxical septal motion. However, the M-mode findings are not specific for an ASD but simply indicate right ventricular volume overload which can occur with other abnormalities such as partial anomalous pulmonary venous drainage and tricuspid or pulmonary regurgitation. Thus it is essential to use the two-dimensional echocardiogram to try to demonstrate the ASD, and while conducting the examination remember that the defect is not always the classical secundum type but can be in the sinus venosus or coronary sinus positions. Where there is doubt as to the site, contrast echocardiography may be of assistance in defining it. The correct diagnosis can be reached in all but a few patients and since pulmonary hypertension rarely occurs in an ASD in childhood, they can be sent for surgical closure without further investigations.

Thus Doppler is of limited value in most patients with an ASD. However, it may be of help in the assessment of the patient with an ASD in several ways: the site may be demonstrated or confirmed from flow across the atrial septum shown with pulsed Doppler or colour flow mapping; an idea of the shunt size, if not exact quantitation, can be obtained from the tricuspid velocity or measurement of right and left-sided volume flow; and associated stenotic or regurgitant lesions can be excluded.

Technique

Following echocardiography Doppler should first be used in an attempt to demonstrate the presence of an ASD and measure the velocity of flow across the atrial septum. For practical purposes an imaging transducer is necessary. It is placed in a subcostal or low parasternal position as would be used for imaging the defect and the echocardiographic image is adjusted to align the transducer as closely as possible to right angles to the septum. The sample volume is placed at the site of echo dropout and as necessary the beam swept along the septum; the scanning plane should also be tilted to image different parts of the septum to ensure maximum flow velocity is obtained or, when no flow is recorded, to be sure that there is none and thus no apparent ASD. The flow signal shows two peaks, one in late systole and the other in late diastole, just after atrial contraction, and often followed by a brief period of flow reversal at the onset of systole (*Figure 8.5*). The

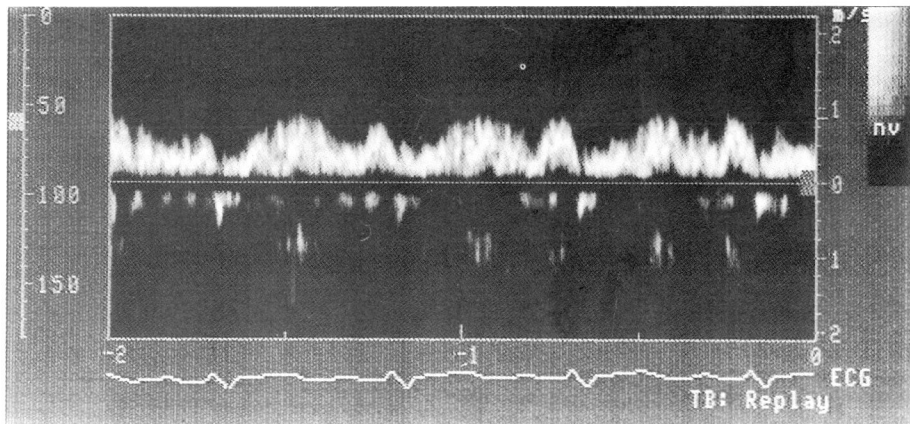

Figure 8.5 Doppler recording through the atrial septal defect from a patient with a significant shunt. The highest velocities occur in systole and immediately following atrial contraction

pulsed Doppler technique provides an accurate means of confirming that an area of echo dropout does represent an ASD. This can be performed more easily, though not necessarily more accurately, using colour Doppler (*see Plate 15*) to demonstrate flow through the defect. A rough estimate of the shunt size can be obtained from the colour image from the breadth and extent of the velocity disturbance through the ASD.

The flow velocity across the tricuspid, pulmonary and mitral valves should also be measured. In the normal subject, the tricuspid maximum velocity is usually less than the mitral but is increased in the presence of an atrial shunt and when this is significant it will usually exceed that through the mitral; the ratio of these gives a further rough estimate of the shunt size[9]. Alternatively the QP/QS can be calculated by using the velocity and area method to measure pulmonary arterial and aortic flow.

If the pulmonary velocity is increased sufficiently to suggest possible valve stenosis, the simple modified Bernoulli formula should not be used to calculate gradient since the increase may just be the result of increased flow. The velocity in the subvalve area is measured; if it is normal there may well be valve stenosis, but if increased to approximately the distal velocity, there is no true valve stenosis. The pulmonary and tricuspid regions are also examined to exclude significant regurgitation as a cause of right ventricular volume overload.

Clinical application

When all findings fit with the diagnosis and echocardiography shows M-mode and two-dimensional evidence of an ASD with a significant shunt, catheterization is not required before surgery. Doppler is worth performing to confirm flow through the defect and exclude associated pulmonary stenosis or more than trivial tricuspid regurgitation. In assessing the gradient across the pulmonary outflow, the velocity in the subvalve area must be taken into account to prevent overestimation due to the increased flow producing an increased velocity over the valve.

An estimate of shunt size from the ratio of tricuspid and mitral velocities or quantitation of QP/QS with Doppler can indicate a moderate or large shunt. However, the M-mode study will indicate a significant shunt and, indeed, if beyond infancy the right ventricular dimension is normal the shunt is so small that surgery is unlikely to be required. Since shunt quantitation is time consuming and impractical as a routine for a busy department it should be preserved for difficult cases; it simply gives a value for the QP/QS and provides no further information on site of the shunt. This may be of some value when an ASD occurs as part of a more complex lesion, but otherwise has little practical application.

It is possible that Doppler may have its most useful role in the assessment of the ASD in determining its site in cases where echocardiography shows right ventricular volume overload, but an ASD cannot be clearly shown. In this context colour Doppler is likely to be the most simple technique; it will show the site of flow through the septum but if it is not available conventional pulsed Doppler with imaging will serve the same purpose and demonstrate left to right flow. Where there appears to be a significant left to right shunt but no evidence of an ASD on echocardiography or Doppler, the diagnosis of partial anomalous pulmonary venous drainage can be assumed and depending on the surgeon's preference catheterization may be indicated. If a pulmonary vein enters the superior vena cava the flow velocity at the junction with the right atrium will be increased and colour Doppler can better demonstrate the junction.

In the partial atrioventricular defect (ostium primum ASD) there is no doubt as to the diagnosis on echocardiography and pulmonary hypertension is uncommon in the absence of a complete atrioventricular defect. Doppler can be used to search for flow from a possible ventricular component, and mitral regurgitation which is a common accompaniment due to abnormal mitral valve morphology. However, the presence of these does not alter the need for surgery or the surgical approach and technique.

Coarctation of the aorta

The care of patients with coarctation generally presents two distinct clinical problems depending on the age of presentation which, in turn is usually related to the anatomical abnormality. In the older infant, child or adult the coarctation is postductal with no ductus arteriosus, while in the newborn infant it is usually preductal, often with ductal flow occurring from the pulmonary artery to the distal aorta. For practical purposes it is appropriate to consider each separately.

Older children

Older patients with coarctation are characteristically asymptomatic, the lesion being recognized by the presence of abnormal femoral pulses, often after a murmur has raised the question of heart disease. In theory, the diagnosis is easily made by clinical examination and most cases are recognized in childhood. Prompt recognition and relief of coarctation are important as the longer the delay in surgery the greater the risks of residual systemic hypertension. However, in a few individuals the condition is missed and they present later, even into adult life, with hypertension or heart failure.

Palpation will, as a rule, allow the diagnosis to be made by the demonstration of weak or delayed femoral pulses; if there is doubt measurement of arm and leg blood pressures with a sphygmomanometer should show a lower blood pressure in the leg than the arm. With few exceptions subsequent investigations are used to demonstrate the site, nature and severity of the obstruction to allow the correct surgical approach. Evidence of rib notching on chest X-ray or left ventricular hypertrophy on ECG are of little practical help since under these circumstances the lesion is likely to be severe and thus clinically evident; they may, however, be incidental findings on investigations performed for other purposes and indicate the need for careful examination of the pulses. Echocardiography from the suprasternal notch can frequently show the narrow segment with post-stenotic dilatation, but the images are generally poorer the older the patient. Thus another means of demonstrating the site of obstruction would be useful and could assist in establishing the diagnosis where there is clinical doubt. By comparison, the assessment of the severity of coarctation of the aorta from pressure drop across it is of relatively little importance since the clinician really only needs to determine that it is present and demonstrate its site to allow prompt and effective surgery.

The most important role of Doppler in the management of the patient with coarctation is likely to be the provision of additional information on the site of the narrowing or the severity of the obstruction.

Technique

The evaluation of coarctation of the aorta with Doppler is generally based on the demonstration of flow disturbance or velocity increase in the distal arch. The blood velocities in the ascending and descending aorta are generally approximately equal, less than 2 m/s and confirmation of the diagnosis with Doppler is most simply based on the demonstration of a normal velocity in the ascending aorta with an increase in the distal arch[11]. An imaging transducer is positioned in the suprasternal notch and adjusted to show the ascending aorta, arch and, if possible, coarctation.

The sample volume should be placed centrally in the ascending aorta and then moved to the proximal arch to obtain their flow velocities which should be similar and within normal limits (*see* Chapter 3). The sample volume is then moved to track flow in the distal arch to just beyond the coarctation site; a flow disturbance will confirm the site while high PRF or continuous wave Doppler will usually be required to measure the maximum velocity (*Figure 8.6*). However, although echocardiography may show the site of the obstruction and suggest optimal angles and sites for obtaining the best signals, continuous wave Doppler should always be used to determine the best signal and imaging is not necessarily required. A stand alone probe can be placed in the suprasternal notch and angled downwards to give optimal flow up the ascending aorta and when it is tilted to the left and posteriorly to obtain flow in the distal arch the increased velocity signal in coarctation is usually readily picked up. Occasionally a higher velocity signal is obtained from a high left parasternal position. If possible an imaging transducer (or careful clinical examination) should be used as signals similar to those in coarctation can be recorded from the same position in patients with left pulmonary artery stenosis.

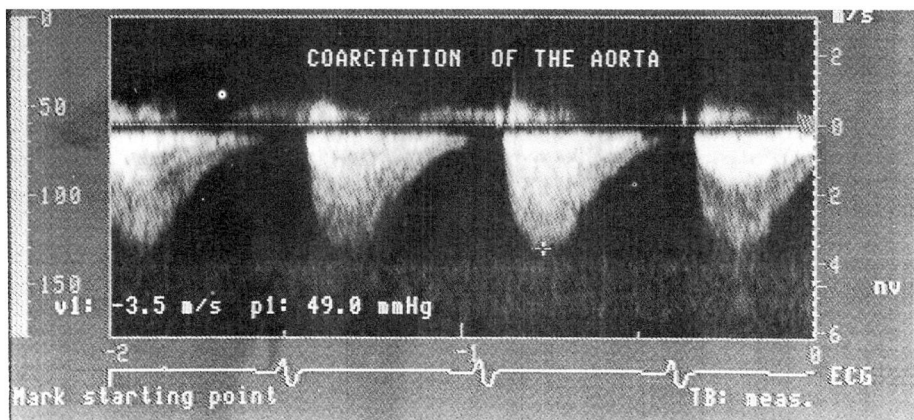

Figure 8.6 Continuous wave recording of flow in the distal aortic arch from the suprasternal notch from a patient with coarctation of the aorta. The maximum velocity of 3.5 m/s (gradient 49 mmHg) is superimposed on a lower velocity signal (2 m/s) from a proximal position

    The maximal flow velocity signal obtained from patients with coarctation shows a variety of waveforms. The maximum velocity always occurs in systole while the diastolic flow varies in different patients; it is generally of low velocity and may not be recognized if the high pass filter is set too high. Thus, in studying a patient with suspected coarctation not only should the highest velocity signal be obtained, but the high pass filter should be adjusted and if necessary reduced to try to show diastolic flow. In the majority, flow continues with low velocity throughout diastole, while in others it occurs only in early diastole or, in a few, is confined entirely to systole. The presence of diastolic flow to some extent reflects the diastolic pressure difference but this will vary with the patient's age and the presence of collateral vessels and in itself is not related to the severity of narrowing. The continuous wave signal can show superimposition of the lower velocity signal from the arch proximal to the coarctation.
    When the Doppler gradient is calculated from the simple modified Bernoulli equation and the maximum velocity, comparison of this with the measured one has shown a poor correlation with both over and underestimation[11] and for the present this should not be used as an indication of the severity of the anatomic; obstruction. Indeed, in the more severe cases there may be so little flow through the obstruction that a Doppler signal cannot be obtained; on occasions in this situation, flow towards the suprasternal notch through a collateral artery may be shown as continuous flow with maximal velocity in systole and low diastolic levels. The poor correlation may result from angulation problems with Doppler (causing underestimation) or, more likely, from difficulties with accurate pressure measurement at catheterization, including the difference between the peak-to-peak and instantaneous gradients. The velocity in the arch proximal to the coarctation should theoretically be included in the calculation of gradient; failure to do this can cause overestimation of, for instance, 4 mmHg for 1.0 m/s and 16 mmHg for 2.0 m/s. In general, a velocity of greater than 2.5 m/s is found in patients with coarctation but higher values may be found in patients in whom the anatomical obstruction is not sufficiently severe to warrant surgical intervention.

Clinical application

The practical value of Doppler in coarctation is best considered under its two different uses: (1) the confirmation of the presence and demonstration of the site of coarctation; and (2) assessment of its severity.

Doppler can assist in the diagnosis of doubtful cases of coarctation by the demonstration of an increased flow velocity (>2.5 m/s) from the distal arch, while that in the ascending aorta is virtually normal. Tracking flow with pulsed or high PRF Doppler demonstrates increased velocity at or just below the site of narrowing. However, failure to show this increased velocity does not necessarily mean there is no coarctation and if no signal away from the transducer is obtained the obstruction may be extremely severe and in the presence of clinical coarctation indicates the need for invasive studies.

Where echocardiography does not give a clear anatomical demonstration of the narrowing colour Doppler flow mapping may add to the use of pulsed or high PRF in its localization. Often the impression of narrowing and poststenotic dilatation is obtained on echocardiography from older patients, but the image is not of diagnostic quality; colour Doppler may enhance the image of the narrowed segment and better outline the area of poststenotic dilatation.

Doppler may theoretically be of value by assessing the pressure drop across the obstruction when accurate measurement of arm and leg blood pressures is difficult. It is important to realize that clinical examination indicates delay in the pressure wave or difference in pulse pressures which is related not just to the severity of the obstruction, but also to collateral flow and is different from the measurement of the systolic pressure difference with Doppler. Thus peripheral pulse volumes may be very different while the systolic pressures are relatively close.

Since Doppler estimation of pressure drop has shown poor correlation with the measured one and exact pressure measurement is not important in comparison to the anatomical demonstration of the severity of obstruction, Doppler measurement of pressure gradient must not in itself be used to assess the need for coarctation surgery. Some evidence suggests that comparison of pressure gradient may be more accurate in postoperative patients where obstruction will be mild and collateral flow of little significance[12].

Experience suggests that outside the neonatal period a velocity from the distal arch of less than 2.5 m/s is unlikely to be associated with significant coarctation, but one of greater than 3 m/s is almost always significant and requiring operation. However, Doppler is not of clear discriminatory value in the range 2.5–3.5 m/s which can be found in both those who do and those who do not require surgical treatment.

The Doppler signals can show considerable variation and with increasing severity it has been suggested that the duration of the signal will increase and, in particular, flow will continue throughout diastole. However, this pattern will depend not only on the severity of the lesion but also the presence of collateral arteries which are not found in young patients but develop with age. The diastolic velocity does, indeed, indicate the pressure difference across the coarctation site but this in itself is not really of clinical value.

Newborn infant

In the newborn infant coarctation is usually preductal and its management is the field of the specialist paediatric cardiologist and surgeon. The presentation and diagnostic features are complicated by the presence of a ductus arteriosus distal to the obstruction and vary depending upon its degree of patency. These infants usually present with cardiac failure and poor femoral pulses, but even with complete arch obstruction if the duct is widely patent flow from the pulmonary artery to descending aorta may be such that there is no clinical difference between the arm and leg pulses. Chest X-ray typically shows cardiomegaly and pulmonary oedema but no features specifically indicating coarctation, and the ECG shows right with little left ventricular hypertrophy.

Echocardiography can demonstrate the ascending aorta, the arch and proximal descending aorta and, in coarctation, usually provides images of the obstruction of diagnostic quality allowing the correct diagnosis and surgical approach to be undertaken. Should a clear demonstration of the obstruction not be obtained, the thoracic and abdominal aorta is examined for lack of pulsation (suggesting a proximal obstruction) and imaged for a distal coarctation. Under these circumstances Doppler may theoretically be of assistance in confirming the presence and site of a coarctation. However, the ductus arteriosus leads from the pulmonary artery directly to the descending aorta and joins it just distal to the typical site for a preductal coarctation; blood can flow through the coarctation from the proximal to distal aorta but, if the arch obstruction is severe and the ductus arteriosus is open, blood will also flow from the pulmonary artery to the descending aorta in a very similar direction. Thus it may not always be easy to ascertain whether the flow signal is being obtained from the coarctation site or ductus arteriosus.

Technique

Ultrasound studies are best performed from the suprasternal notch or upper left sternal edge in a similar way to older patients. The shape of some imaging transducers can cause problems and a separate Doppler transducer often fits better into the suprasternal notch and gives an improved signal. Continuous wave or high PRF Doppler can show an increased velocity of flow and tracking with pulsed or high PRF Doppler indicates that this occurs just distal to the coarctation site. An attempt to determine whether this is the signal of coarctation or ductal flow should be made, but this can be difficult because of their proximity. In these circumstances it is worth examining the descending thoracic aorta from a subcostal position: by comparison with the ascending aorta there can be a significant difference between the acceleration time and acceleration slope[13] of the flow signal, but there is some overlap and the findings are not diagnostic.

Clinical application

In the newborn infant with coarctation, the flow velocity recorded from the region of the distal arch is, as a rule, less than in older patients, frequently in the range 2.2–2.8 m/s (equivalent to approximately 20–30 mmHg). However, because of the proximity of the coarctation and mouth of the ductus, even with an imaging system, it is not always possible to ascertain whether this is ductal or aortic flow. Thus an increased velocity signal may indicate flow through a coarctation or ductus arteriosus. It may be interpreted as indicating arch obstruction but not necessarily coarctation as it may also be found in arch interruption with a restrictive ductus.

Prostaglandin infusion by opening the ductus arteriosus may result in a fall in the maximal velocity of this signal (*Figure 8.7*) and Doppler study of the newborn

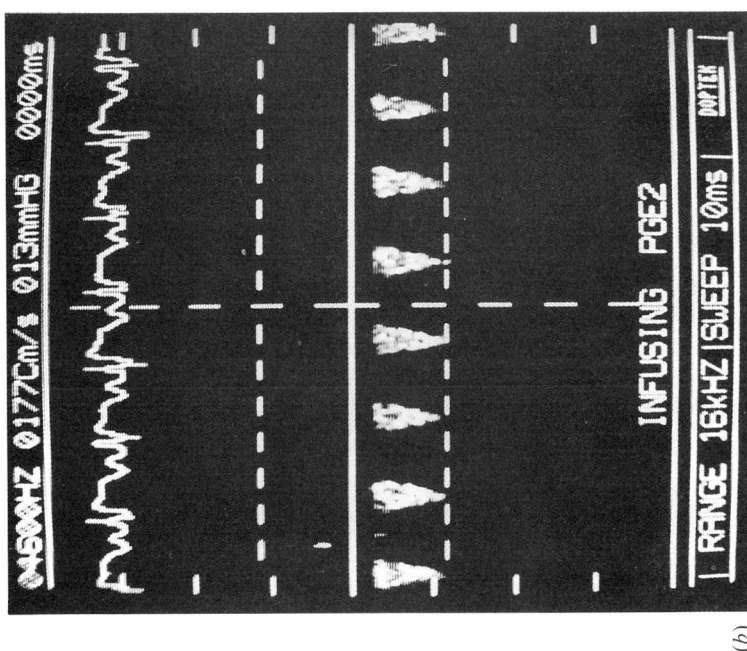

(a)

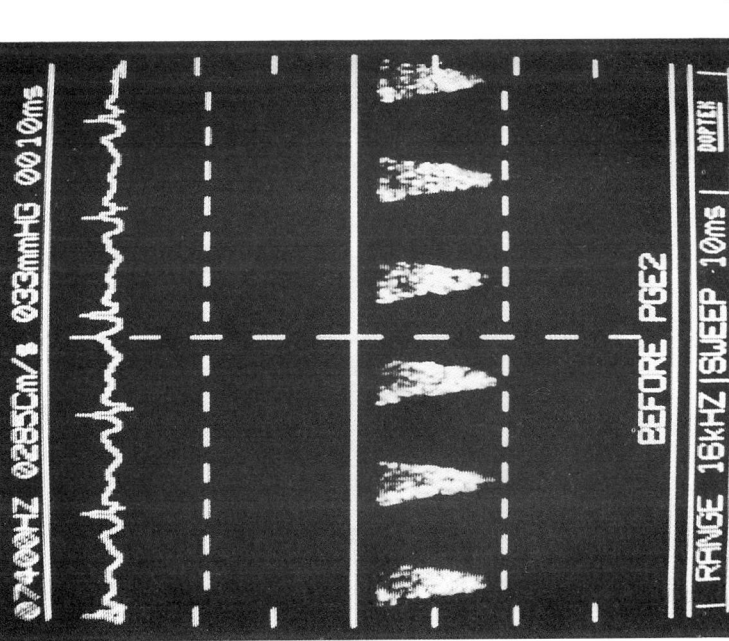

(b)

Figure 8.7 Continuous wave recording from a newborn infant with coarctation of the aorta. The transducer is positioned in the suprasternal notch and angled towards the distal aortic arch: the initial signal (*a*) has a maximum velocity of 2.85 m/s but after infusion of prostaglandins (*b*) this has fallen to 1.77 m/s, suggesting that ductal flow has been recorded

infant on prostaglandins may show no increased velocity even in the presence of very severe obstruction or interruption. As a corollary, the abolition of an increased velocity with prostaglandin indicates a lower pressure in the distal aorta than pulmonary artery and, in the context of an infant with possible aortic obstruction, would be likely to confirm severe obstruction, either coarctation or interrupted arch. However, similar information can of course also be obtained from palpation of the femoral pulses.

There is usually little doubt as to the presence of a coarctation and the surgeon simply requires the demonstration of its anatomical site and nature. Thus Doppler is of limited value in assessing the newborn infant with suspected coarctation, and clinical examination and echocardiography remain the main non-invasive investigations. However, the use of colour Doppler to enhance the images of the site of narrowing, and differentiate aortic from ductal flow, may well prove to be important in difficult cases.

Innocent murmur

The paediatric cardiologist, general paediatrician and adult physician are frequently referred asymptomatic patients who may have an innocent murmur. In this situation it is important to make a firm diagnosis of an innocent murmur as opposed to a mild cardiac defect in order to give clear and definite reassurance to the patient or parents, and discharge the patient without recommending antibiotic prophylaxis against infective endocarditis. These patients will be asymptomatic and the murmur is usually one of the classical innocent ones but, on occasions, there may be some doubt as to this. In particular, the question may arise as to whether there is a mitral valve abnormality, a small VSD, an ASD or mild pulmonary stenosis, or mild aortic stenosis rather than a carotid bruit.

The ECG will be normal in mild lesions (although a significant ASD is unlikely in the absence of an rsR') and the chest X-ray unhelpful. Similarly echocardiography may show an abnormal aortic or mitral valve or an ASD, but can equally well be normal without excluding a mild abnormality. In these circumstances Doppler is extremely valuable and indeed, with the exception of the ASD, probably the most appropriate of the non-invasive techniques.

The Doppler examination should be designed to measure the maximum velocity over all four valves and seek an abnormal degree of regurgitation, bearing in mind that right-sided valve regurgitation is a normal finding and not an indication for more investigation or follow-up, or for antibiotic prophylaxis against infective endocarditis. A VSD jet should then be sought with continuous wave or colour Doppler. The jet through a small lesion may occur for only part of systole and can sometimes be difficult to record easily and quickly, and particular care is needed before saying it is absent when the murmur is in the typical site of a VSD.

An occasional difficulty can occur when a measured velocity is just outside the normal quoted range. If all other factors indicate no cardiac abnormality, it is the present author's practice to consider this a variant of normal and dismiss the child from follow-up: if there is a very mild lesion it is not likely to cause problems and routine reassessment is unnecessary. On the other hand, the documentation of a lesion such as a small VSD or mild pulmonary stenosis allows a rational explanation to be given and follow-up will depend on individual practice.

Doppler is of considerable assistance in assessing these patients but, on occasions, it will raise more problems due to unexpected findings. Thus ductal flow or mitral regurgitation can be shown when there is no murmur typical of these lesions, and flow through a tiny ASD may be found where the right ventricular size is normal and thus the shunt is very small. Since these lesions would not have been recognized in the past it seems appropriate to take no action under these circumstances and long-term follow-up does not seem necessary. However, although it has been said that infective endocarditis can occur in patients with normal hearts this raises the question as to whether these patients may have a very minor unrecognized abnormality.

As with echocardiography it is of course mandatory that any physician ordering this investigation has a clear understanding of the pitfalls of the investigation in order that the decision on clinical management is made on the basis of all the information available and not just on the ultrasound studies which, useful as they are, are not infallible since performance and interpretation are only as good as the operator performing them.

References

1. BARRON, J. V., SAHN, D. J., VALDES-CRUZ, L. M. *et al.* (1984) Clinical utility of two-dimensional Doppler echocardiographic techniques for estimating pulmonary to systemic blood flow ratios in children with left to right shunting atrial septal defect, ventricular septal defect or patent ductus arteriosus. *J. Am. Coll. Cardiol*, **3**, 169–178
2. SUTHERLAND, G. R., GODMAN, M. J., SMALLHORN, J. F., GUITERRAS, P., ANDERSON, R. H. and HUNTER, S. (1982) Ventricular septal defects. Two-dimensional echocardiographic and morphological correlations. *Br. Heart J.*, **47**, 316–328
3. STEVENSON, J. G., KABORAWI, I., DOOLEY, T. and GUNTHOROTH, W. G. (1978) Diagnosis of ventricular septal defect by pulsed Doppler echocardiography. *Circulation*, **58**, 322–326
4. HATLE, L. and ANGELSEN, B. (1985) *Doppler Ultrasound in Cardiology: Physical Principles and Clinical Applications*, 2nd edn, pp. 236–252. Philadelphia: Lea and Febiger
5. MURPHY, D. J., LUDOMIRSKY, A. and HUHTA, J. C. (1986) Continuous wave Doppler in children with ventricular septal defect: noninvasive estimation of interventricular pressure gradient. *Am. J. Cardiol.*, **57**, 428–432
6. LUDOMIRSKY, A., HUHTA, J. C., VICK, G. W., MURPHY, D. J., DANFORD, D. A., MORROW, W. R. (1986) Color Doppler detection of multiple ventricular septal defects. *Circulation*, **74**, 1317–1322
7. STEVENSON, J. G., KAWABORI, I. and GUNTHOROTH, W. G. (1979) Noninvasive detection of pulmonary hypertension in patent ductus arteriosus by pulsed Doppler echocardiography. *Circulation*, **60**, 355–359
8. HATLE, L. and ANGELSEN, B. (1985) *Doppler Ultrasound in Cardiology: Physical Principles and Clinical Applications*, 2nd edn, pp. 220–228. Philadelphia: Lea and Febiger
9. HATLE, L. and ANGELSEN, B. (1985) *Doppler Ultrasound in Cardiology: Physical Principles and Clinical Applications*, 2nd edn, pp. 234–235. Philadelphia: Lea and Febiger
10. HATLE, L. and ANGELSEN, B. (1985) *Doppler Ultrasound in Cardiology: Physical Principles and Clinical Applications*, 2nd edn, pp. 217–220. Philadelphia: Lea and Febiger
11. HOUSTON, A. B., SIMPSON, I. A., POLLOCK, J. C. S., JAMIESON, M. P. G., DOIG, W. B. and COLEMAN, E. N. (1987) Doppler ultrasound in the assessment of severity of coarctation of the aorta and interruption of the aortic arch obstruction. *Br. Heart J.*, **57**, 38–43
12. WYSE, R. K. H., ROBINSON, P. J., DEANFIELD, J. E. and TUNSTALL-PEDOE, D. S. (1984) Use of continuous wave Doppler ultrasound velocimetry to assess the severity of coarctation of the aorta by measurement of aortic flow velocities. *Br. Heart J.*, **52**, 278–283
13. SHADDY, R. E., SUIDEF, A. R., SILVERMAN, N. H. and LUTIN, W. (1986) Pulsed Doppler findings in patients with coarctation of the aorta. *Circulation*, **73**, 82–88

9

Prosthetic valve function

Iain A. Simpson

Clinical assessment of the patient with a prosthetic valve replacement is of considerable importance but is often difficult, particularly when both the mitral and aortic valves have been replaced. Under these circumstances a systolic murmur is often associated with an aortic valve prosthesis, especially when this is relatively small, and can mask or sometimes mimic the presence of mitral prosthetic regurgitation. Although prosthetic valve malfunction is often manifest by symptomatic deterioration, the contribution of other factors such as left ventricular dysfunction, irreversible pulmonary hypertension or coexistent pulmonary disease can complicate any clinical assessment.

Echocardiography can be extremely useful in the investigation of these patients, both in identifying structural abnormalities of the valve prosthesis and in assessing chamber dimensions and ventricular function. Where a significant structural abnormality is found at echocardiography, major prosthetic malfunction is invariably present, but echocardiography remains a relatively insensitive technique for detecting prosthetic malfunction, and cannot therefore exclude its presence with any certainty[1]. The problems are compounded in patients with a mechanical prosthesis where the dense pyrolite and steel structures cause distortion of ultrasound data used in the construction of echocardiographic images, resulting from the fact that assumptions of the properties of ultrasound in biological tissue are not valid for mechanical prostheses. Occasionally, however, inferences regarding mechanical valve malfunction can be made from echocardiography, but the frequency with which this is possible has not made a major clinical impact on the assessment of these patients. The value of radiographic screening of radiopaque mechanical prostheses should not be forgotten, but again, difficulties can arise in obtaining an adequate profile of the valve, and the presence of pannus or clot formation may cause obstruction of a mechanical prosthesis without any apparent abnormality of valve motion at screening.

Accurate haemodynamic information is of critical importance in the assessment of a patient with suspected prosthetic valve malfunction but cannot be provided by either echocardiography or cardiac screening and thus many patients require cardiac catheterization. Although accepted as a routine procedure, this is not entirely free from risk, and this is increased by the fact that many patients with prosthetic valves, and all with mechanical prostheses, are on long-term anticoagulant therapy. In addition, cardiac catheterization is not always successful in obtaining the necessary haemodynamic information in these patients. Thus, the presence of a mechanical aortic prosthesis or of vegetations in prosthetic endocarditis make it impossible to enter the left ventricular cavity safely and angiography cannot then be performed to assess the presence and extent of mitral regurgitation. Furthermore, the induction of ventricular tachycardia during angiography can produce a degree of mitral regurgitation in a normally competent valve, though this should rarely cause confusion with a significant regurgitant lesion.

Clearly, the non-invasive assessment of cardiac haemodynamics now possible with Doppler ultrasound, has been a major development in the investigation of patients with suspected prosthetic valve malfunction. If Doppler ultrasound is to be of extensive clinical value in this area it must be a valid technique for both bioprosthetic and mechanical prostheses, be able to identify normal prosthetic valve function and distinguish this from significant prosthetic obstruction, determine accurately the presence of prosthetic regurgitation and, if possible, provide some assessment as to its severity.

Normal prosthetic valve flow

The presence of any artificial valve, even when functioning normally, confers a degree of obstruction to blood flow and a small but non-significant gradient can be measured across both mechanical and bioprosthetic valves *in vivo*[2, 3]. An increase in the flow velocity measured by Doppler ultrasound would therefore be expected across normally functioning prostheses as opposed to native valves (*see* Chapter 3). Similarly, for normally functioning mitral prostheses a slightly prolonged mitral pressure half-time would be expected. The range of peak flow velocities and pressure half-times differs slightly between prostheses of different types. Although all mechanical prostheses have an inherent trivial degree of regurgitation, it is rarely possible to identify this in a normally functioning mitral prosthesis because of the poor ultrasound transmission through these structures which produces a small area immediately behind the mechanical structure from which information cannot be obtained. This is not the case in patients with an aortic mechanical valve replacement, where continuous wave Doppler from the apical position may identify trivial regurgitation in a significant proportion of patients with normally functioning prostheses[4]. This indicates the sensitivity of Doppler and does not necessarily denigrate its value in assessing the presence of significant valve regurgitation in these patients. Although all bioprosthetic valves have a minor regurgitant volume associated with initial closure of the valve, it is not normal for Doppler to detect the presence of regurgitation through a tissue prosthesis after the valve has closed. With the exception of an aortic Bjork–Shiley prosthesis, therefore, the presence of regurgitation through any prosthetic valve detected by continuous wave Doppler ultrasound should be regarded as abnormal.

Mitral valve prostheses

Doppler ultrasound examination of a mitral prosthesis, as for normal mitral flow and mitral stenosis, is best performed with the patient in the left lateral position and the transducer at the apex from where it is almost always possible to identify mitral prosthetic flow. Flow through a mitral prosthesis can occasionally be directed more anteriorly than normal, particularly with a mechanical disc prosthesis, and the optimal Doppler signal, and occasionally the only signal, is sometimes obtained

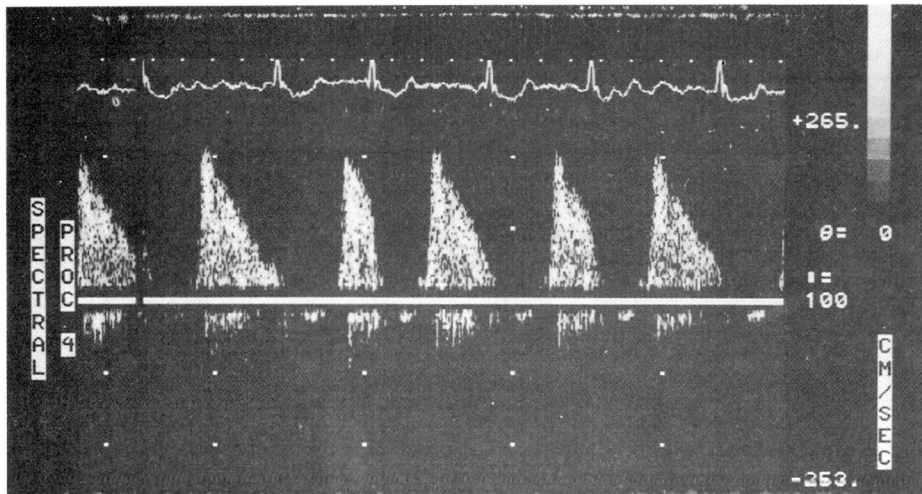

Figure 9.1 Continuous wave Doppler spectral display of diastolic mitral flow velocity across a normally functioning mitral prosthesis. Note the loss of a second velocity peak with the patient in atrial fibrillation

from the lower left sternal edge rather than the apex. The appearance of normal mitral prosthetic flow is similar to that through native valves, demonstrating the biphasic flow velocity pattern resulting from atrial contraction. However, few patients with a mitral prosthesis remain in sinus rhythm, the vast majority being in sustained atrial fibrillation where no second velocity peak occurs (*Figure 9.1*).

Mechanical valve prostheses produce characteristic high intensity clicks associated with both opening and closure (*Figure 9.2*). These high amplitude signals close to the mitral prosthetic flow can mask a flow signal of low intensity, but can also be valuable in the timing of flow velocity recordings, in particular distinguishing mitral regurgitation from aortic stenosis. Since the signal associated with opening of a mechanical mitral prosthesis is close to the initial peak velocity on

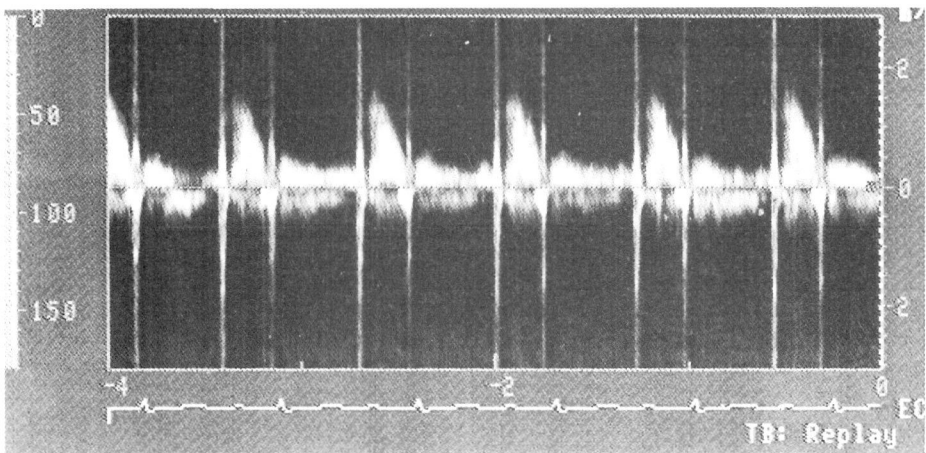

Figure 9.2 Discrete high intensity valve 'clicks' associated with opening and closure of a mechanical mitral valve replacement

the spectral recording it can produce the impression of a falsely high peak velocity, although the true peak can usually be identified by careful examination of the spectrum.

Flow through a competent prosthesis will be determined by the cardiac output and the peak mitral velocity will vary with both the size and type of prosthesis and with the pressure drop between the left atrium and left ventricle at the beginning of diastole. The normal range of peak flow velocities for a variety of prosthetic valves without evidence of regurgitation is shown in *Table 9.1*. Similar results for porcine valves have been reported[5]. Mitral prostheses with regurgitation will have an

Table 9.1 Peak velocities across mitral prostheses (m/s)

Type	Range	Mean
Bjork–Shiley	1.10–1.85	1.52
Carpentier–Edwards	1.22–1.68	1.44
Wessex porcine	1.16–1.66	1.41
Low profile Ionescu–Shiley	1.19–1.47	1.33
Hancock pericardial	1.24–1.78	1.51
St Jude	1.12–1.75	1.35

increase in the diastolic flow and thus an increase in the maximum flow velocity recording. This increase in diastolic flow velocity can prove valuable in confirming the presence of mitral prosthetic regurgitation, particularly when severe[5, 6]. Although the peak velocity will tend to be higher the smaller the prosthesis, the range of valve diameters inserted tends to be narrow for a particular type of mitral prosthesis and, since the diastolic pressure drop is relatively low, this would appear to be of little relevance.

It can be seen from *Table 9.1* that, in many instances, the peak flow velocity will be within the range that pulsed Doppler is able to measure accurately without the occurrence of frequency aliasing. This will produce a much 'cleaner' Doppler spectral signal, the Doppler sample gate being positioned within the velocity jet and excluding the low velocity signals picked up along the Doppler beam by continuous wave examination. However, even with a normally functioning mitral prosthesis the peak flow velocity can exceed the Nyquist limit and frequency aliasing can occur. Since the maximum velocity curve and peak velocity will be identical on continuous and pulsed Doppler, where the latter is possible without aliasing, there seems little benefit of using pulsed Doppler for practical clinical purposes, since searching for the optimal mitral flow velocity recording by continuous wave examination allows quicker and easier identification of the velocity pattern of mitral prosthetic flow, particularly when using a stand alone Doppler system.

Validity of Bernoulli equation

In Chapter 5, the modified Bernoulli equation was applied to the maximum flow velocity curve in patients with mitral valve disease, and the validity of using this equation in these patients has been established in both the measurement of mitral valve gradients and the estimation of the mitral pressure half-time. Although of value in assessing native mitral valve disease, the assumptions necessary to apply this equation may be questioned for valve prostheses. Application of the modified Bernoulli equation to the maximum flow velocity recorded *in vitro* in a pulsatile flow model, and comparison of the Doppler derived pressure gradient with that measured directly, has confirmed that the estimated Doppler gradient is almost identical to that measured directly in the test apparatus[7]. Despite the potential problems and assumptions of using the modified Bernoulli equation to estimate gradients across prosthetic valves, its application remains valid and it is therefore possible to apply Doppler ultrasound *in vivo* to assess valve gradients and pressure half-time in patients with a mitral valve replacement[8].

Calculation of mitral prosthetic gradients

In clinical terms, the peak mitral gradient is of little relevance as mitral gradients at catheterization are usually measured as a mean value over the diastolic time period. Calculation of the peak pressure drop from the peak mitral flow velocity across a prosthetic valve will not therefore relate to a mean gradient as measured at catheterization and, since the relationship between velocity and pressure drop is not linear, averaging the maximum velocity over diastole and applying the modified Bernoulli equation is not valid. As discussed in Chapter 6 the instantaneous pressure drop must be calculated from the maximum velocity at each point throughout diastole, for practical purposes at each 5 or 10 ms interval, and then averaged to estimate the mean prosthetic gradient. When this is carried out the gradients estimated by Doppler ultrasound are fairly accurate when compared with those measured at cardiac catheterization[9–11] for bioprosthetic and mechanical prostheses, whether normal or obstructed and in the presence or absence of prosthetic mitral regurgitation.

The mitral pressure half-time in patients with a mitral valve prosthesis is calculated in an identical way to that used in mitral stenosis and discussed in Chapter 5, although in patients with a mechanical prosthesis difficulties can occasionally arise in accurately identifying the peak velocity because of the proximity of the high amplitude signal associated with opening of the prosthesis. Despite this the measurement of mitral pressure half-time is of considerable value in identifying obstruction of a mitral prosthesis in either the absence or presence of coexisting regurgitation (*see Figures 9.3* and *9.4*).

Mean mitral prosthetic gradients and mitral pressure half-times for a variety of normally functioning valve prostheses are shown in *Table 9.2*. Although

Table 9.2 Mitral pressure half-times and mean valve gradients across mitral prostheses

	Half-time (ms)		Mean gradient (mmHg)	
	Range	*Mean*	*Range*	*Mean*
Bjork–Shiley	40–180	88	0–10	3.6
Carpentier–Edwards	50–160	85	2–14	5.6
Wessex porcine	40–140	82	2.1–6.5	3.6
Low profile Ionescu–Shiley	50–170	82	2.1–8.3	3.4
Hancock pericardial	40–180	98	2.2–8.3	4.2
St Jude	40–160	90	0–8.0	4.5

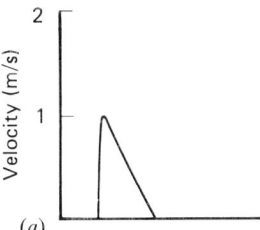
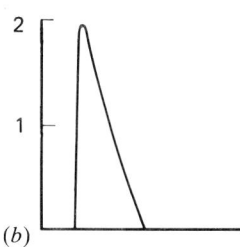
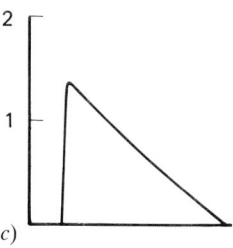

Figure 9.3 Diagram of mitral inflow velocities in atrial fibrillation: (*a*) normally functioning mitral prosthesis; (*b*) non-stenotic mitral prosthesis with increased peak velocity resulting from increased diastolic flow as a consequence of significant mitral regurgitation – note that there is no prolongation of the mitral pressure half-time; (*c*) stenotic mitral prosthesis with increased peak velocity and prolonged mitral pressure half-time

mechanical valves are less obstructive than bioprostheses when tested *in vitro* and pericardial less so than porcine prostheses[12, 13], there is a wide range of mean gradients and pressure half-times *in vivo*, with little differences between various valve types. This illustrates the complex pressure/flow relationships that exist across valve prostheses *in vivo*, and that *in vitro* data cannot always be extrapolated to the clinical situation, highlighting the potential value of Doppler ultrasound in this area.

Mitral prosthetic obstruction

The appearance of mitral bioprosthetic obstruction is identical to that found in mitral stenosis. The peak diastolic flow velocity is usually increased and more importantly the rate at which this velocity decreases is reduced dependent on the severity of obstruction (*Figures 9.3* and *9.4*). This has the effect of both increasing the estimated mean prosthetic gradient and of prolonging the mitral pressure half-time. Obstruction of a bioprosthetic valve can span the whole range of severity from mild obstruction to severe stenosis. Obstruction of a mechanical mitral prosthesis is usually due either to clot or pannus formation and is almost always associated with a dramatic haemodynamic upset. This is usually apparent clinically, with loss of prosthetic clicks noticed either by the patient or on clincial examination. Pulmonary oedema quickly develops and rapid surgical intervention is required. Swift, accurate diagnosis is therefore critical. A 'stuck' mechanical disc prosthesis can often be confirmed by cardiac screening or two-dimensional echocardiography. However, the full profile of the disc, necessary to identify the degree of opening, cannot always be easily obtained by X-ray screening, and where there is a ball-valve type thrombus it is possible for the disc to be tilting normally and for this to be missed by echocardiography. Doppler ultrasound can accurately assess obstruction to mitral blood flow and therefore prove of major clinical value in the assessment of these patients.

Continuous wave Doppler examination in these patients with obstructed mechanical prostheses will produce a high velocity, low intensity spectral signal, with little or no decrease in the maximum mitral flow velocity throughout diastole, i.e. a markedly prolonged or indefinite mitral pressure half-time (*Figure 9.5*). It is easy to underestimate the maximum flow velocity on the spectral display because of the low amplitude signal, particularly if high amplitude prosthetic 'clicks' remain.

116

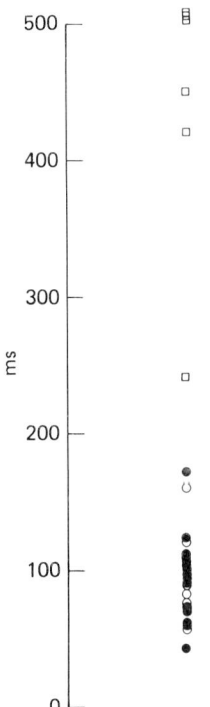

Figure 9.4 Mitral pressure half-time in 32 patients with normal mitral prostheses, mitral prosthetic obstruction and mitral prosthetic regurgitation. Note that the presence of regurgitation does not affect the pressure half-time and those with significant obstruction are easily identified. $n = 32$; ● normal; □ obstructed; ○ regurgitant

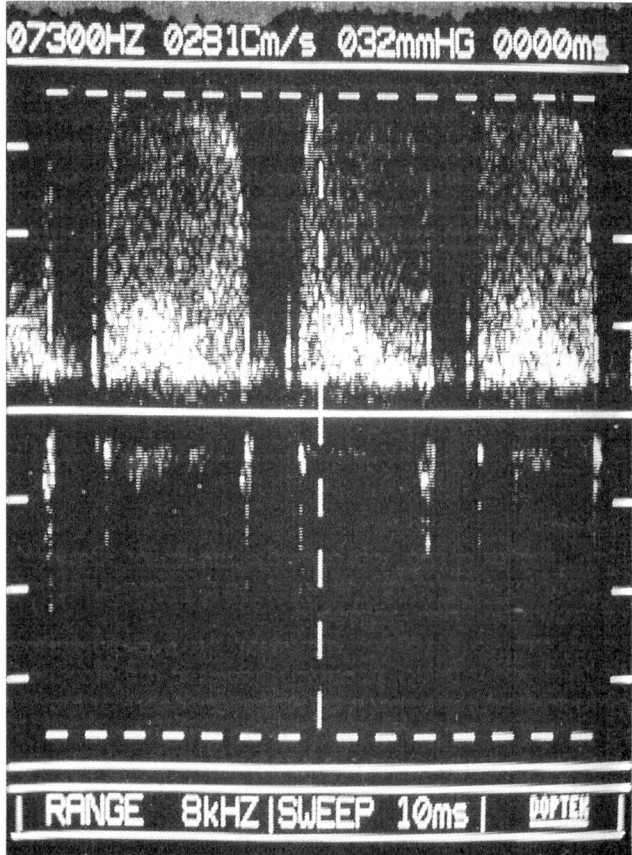

Figure 9.5 Continuous wave Doppler spectral display from patient with an obstructed mechanical mitral valve replacement. Note the onset of flow velocities distinct from aortic valve closure, increased peak velocity and markedly prolonged mitral pressure half-time

However, the discrepancy should be apparent from the high frequency audio signal and appropriate adjustments to the gain settings will usually reveal the high velocity on the spectrum analyser. This problem is well illustrated in *Figure 9.6* in a patient in whom the mechanical disc was sticking only with every second heart beat. When opening normally (arrowed) there was a high intensity, well demarcated signal with an increase in the peak mitral flow velocity, although a relatively normal mitral pressure half-time. During the cardiac cycles when the prosthesis was sticking, however, the very high velocity of the much lower amplitude signal has been masked, but the much prolonged mitral pressure half-time remains apparent. In five patients with obstruction of a mechanical mitral prosthesis, in the present author's experience, rapid confirmation of the prosthetic obstruction was obtained

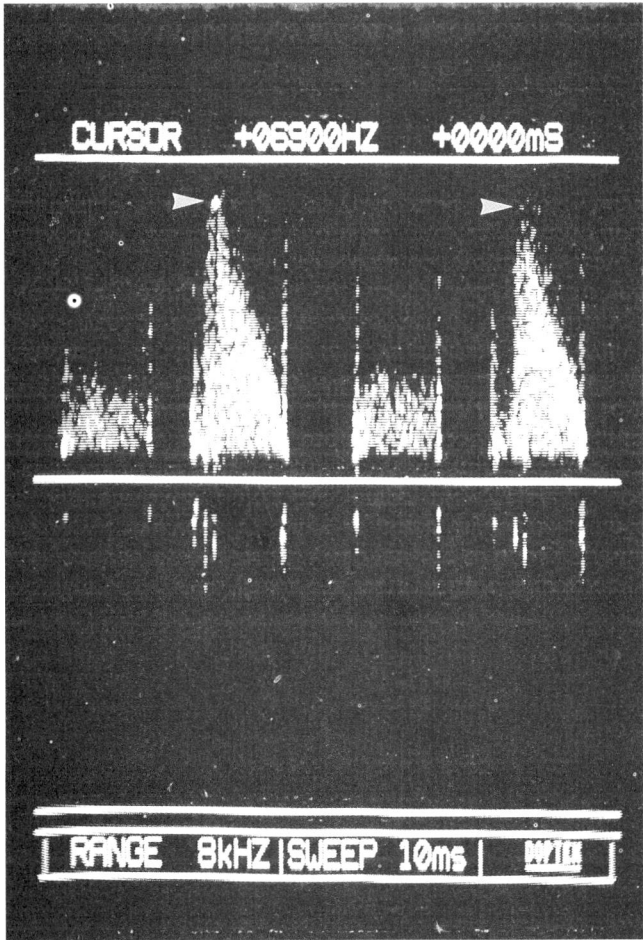

Figure 9.6 Continuous wave Doppler spectral display from patient with Bjork–Shiley mitral valve replacement 'sticking' every second beat. Increased diastolic flow occurring when the valve opens normally (arrowed beats) causes an increase in the peak velocity but relatively normal pressure half-time. In the beats where the valve is sticking the peak velocities are of much lower intensity and not visualized at this gain setting. However, the marked prolongation of the pressure half-time is easily appreciated

by continuous wave Doppler ultrasound examination (*see Figure 9.4*) and three of these patients successfully underwent surgery without further preoperative investigation.

Where sticking of the tilting disc prosthesis is only partial, caused by delay in the initial opening of the valve, the use of pulsed Doppler with simultaneous echo imaging has been reported to show variable timing of the onset of mitral inflow[14].

Aortic valve prostheses

The direction of the jet through a tissue aortic valve replacement will be central in most cases, but less predictable through a mechanical prosthesis. Since the flow direction can be variable, the examination technique required is similar to that for aortic stenosis where multiple precordial positions must be interrogated. In order to align the Doppler beam at an angle which is sufficiently near the line of blood flow, it is necessary to examine the patient from all available praecordial positions (suprasternal, apical, subcostal, right parasternal, supraclavicular) as discussed in Chapter 4. However, in the majority of patients a good Doppler signal will be obtained from the apical position using continuous wave Doppler. With stand alone Doppler the presence of aortic valve clicks in the continuous wave signal is an important marker of flow from the aorta rather than the left ventricular outflow tract. Even where prosthetic valve clicks are present, subtle manipulation of the transducer may be required to identify the optimal signal and the maximum velocity recording.

Calculation of the peak instantaneous aortic prosthetic gradient is, as for other valve lesions, obtained by application of the modified Bernoulli equation to the peak velocity in m/s. It is worth confirming that the velocity proximal to the aortic prosthesis (i.e. that in the left ventricular outflow tract) is not significantly raised; if it is it should be included in the calculation of gradient by the Bernoulli equation (Chapter 2). This is of particular importance in the presence of aortic regurgitation where the systolic velocity of blood in the left ventricular outflow tract may well be elevated and overestimation of the peak aortic prosthetic gradient would occur if this was ignored. Pulsed wave Doppler can easily assess outflow tract flow with the sample volume positioned below the aortic prosthesis from the apical position and will usually be able to measure the peak velocity without aliasing occurring. When this occurs high pulse repetition frequency Doppler can be used, while if it is not available, continuous wave Doppler can almost always provide a satisfactory recording of the left ventricular outflow tract velocity from the apical position by manipulation of the transducer from the mitral flow signal to the aortic signal. Here systolic flow away from the transducer is identified and, in the absence of prosthetic valve clicks, this can be used as a quick check of the proximal velocity in most cases where difficulty is encountered with pulsed wave examination using a duplex scanner.

The range of peak instantaneous aortic gradients calculated from the velocities is shown in *Table 9.3* for a variety of prosthetic valve types in the aortic position. Although there is a tendency for pericardial valves to have lower transvalvar gradients than porcine ones, all aortic prostheses, whether bioprosthetic or mechanical, show a wide range of gradients, this being dependent on cardiac output, ventricular function, prosthetic size and the presence of regurgitation. However, this does not affect the value of serial examinations within an individual patient providing examination conditions are consistent.

Table 9.3 Peak gradients across aortic prostheses

	Gradient (mmHg)	
	Range	Mean
Bjork–Shiley	4–41	19.5
Carpentier–Edwards	12–30	23
Wessex porcine	5–46	20
Low profile Ionescu–Shiley	8–29	16.5
Hancock pericardial	5–27	15
St Jude	7–20	13

Aortic prosthetic obstruction

The assessment of obstruction of a bioprosthetic aortic valve replacement follows the same examination and recording techniques as for aortic stenosis (*see* Chapter 4). Continuous wave Doppler examination from the apical position of a patient with stenosis of an Ionescu–Shiley pericardial xenograft is shown in *Figure 9.7* with a peak instantaneous prosthetic gradient of 170 mmHg.

The presence of significant valve dysfunction is usually suggested by a combination of prosthetic valve degeneration on two-dimensional imaging and the Doppler-derived prosthetic gradient, although echocardiography can appear normal and Doppler examination provide the sole indication of significant aortic prosthetic obstruction[15]. Since aortic valve prostheses are obstructive to a degree even when functioning normally, peak instantaneous aortic prosthetic gradients as

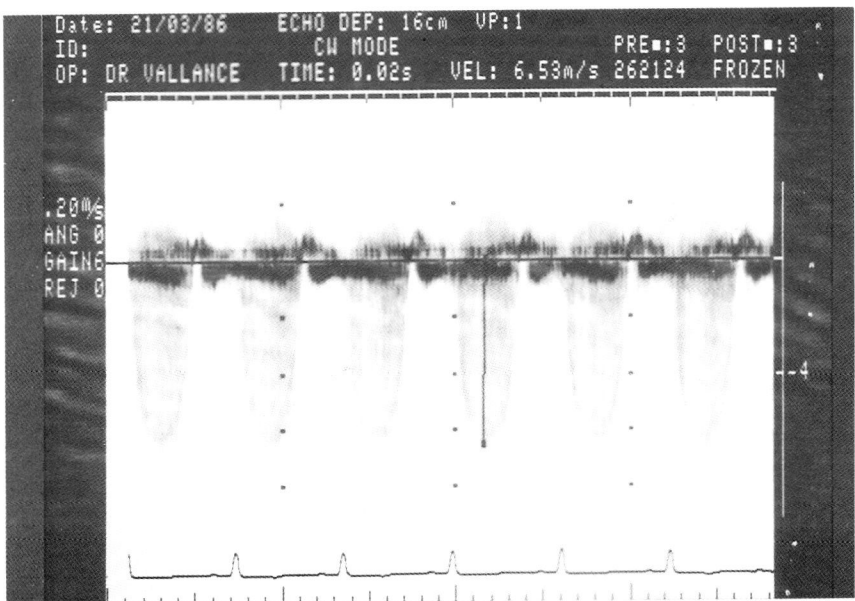

Figure 9.7 Continuous wave Doppler spectral display from apical position of patient with severe stenosis of a bioprosthetic aortic valve replacement, with peak instantaneous pressure gradient calculated as 170 mmHg

high as 40 mmHg should not necessarily be regarded as abnormal in the absence of structural abnormality of the valve prosthesis. It should be remembered that the presence of significant aortic regurgitation, although indicating significant valve dysfunction, will cause an increase in the aortic systolic velocity recording which does not in itself imply stenosis of the prosthesis.

Obstruction or sticking of a mechanical aortic valve prosthesis is a rare but life-threatening situation, requiring rapid surgical intervention. The diagnosis is not usually in doubt and it is usually not difficult to profile adequately the valve with cardiac screening and confirm the diagnosis. The present author has no experience of Doppler ultrasound in this condition and, although a very high velocity jet will be present, the direction of the jet will be completely unpredictable and it may be difficult and time consuming to identify. It may be that Doppler ultrasound will prove of little clinical value in this particular situation.

Tricuspid valve prostheses

Tricuspid valve replacements are uncommon but are easily accessible to assessment by Doppler ultrasound. Doppler examination should be performed as for a normal valve, either from the cardiac apex with the transducer angled to the right in the same plane as mitral flow or from the left parasternal region with the transducer angled under the sternum or from the subcostal position. Patients with a tricuspid valve replacement will almost invariably be in atrial fibrillation.

Assessment of the degree of obstruction of a tricuspid valve replacement is identical to that for mitral valve prostheses. The peak tricuspid flow velocity will vary with respiration but should not exceed 1.5 m/s in a normally functioning, competent tricuspid prosthesis. The degree of prosthetic obstruction can be assessed from the tricuspid pressure half-time, which should not be affected by variation in flow with respiration, and is not usually greater than 100 ms in a normal tricuspid replacement.

Prosthetic valve regurgitation

The assessment of prosthetic valve regurgitation is a far more common clinical problem than prosthetic obstruction and if Doppler ultrasound is to prove valuable in the management of patients with suspected prosthetic valve dysfunction it must be able accurately to identify or exclude the presence of prosthetic valve regurgitation. In addition, the clinical value of the technique would be further enhanced if it were able to provide some assessment of its severity.

Presence of mitral prosthetic regurgitation

Identification of the presence of mitral prosthetic regurgitation is best achieved using continuous wave Doppler examination from the apical position from which the relatively broad Doppler beam, which measures velocities throughout its length, will detect a high velocity, pansystolic jet away from the transducer (*Figure 9.8*). With continuous wave Doppler the detection of significant mitral regurgitation in native valve disease is usually fairly easy if the operator has a reasonable proficiency in the use of cardiac Doppler ultrasound, but this is not always the case with regurgitation through a mitral valve replacement. Both the

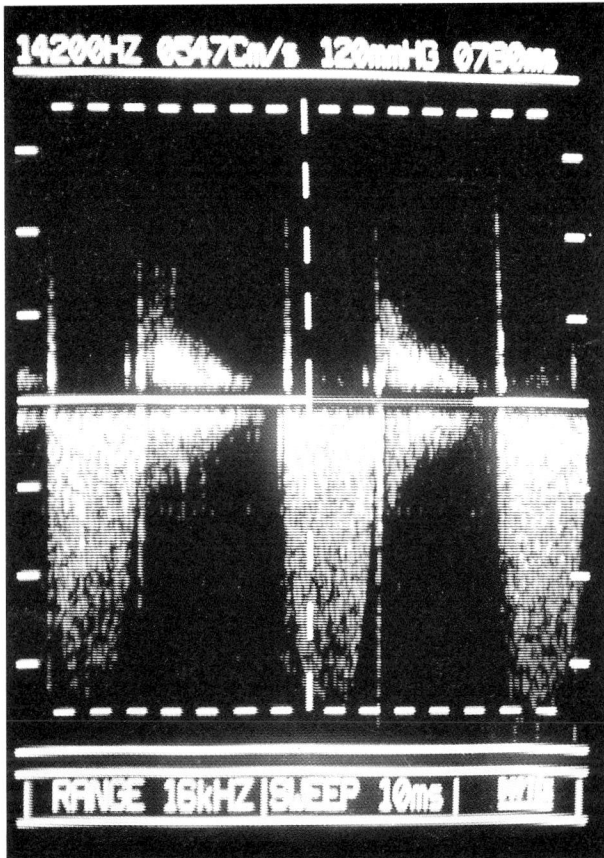

Figure 9.8 Continuous wave Doppler spectral display of prosthetic mitral regurgitation from the apical position. Note the high velocity pansystolic jet with the flow velocity onset occurring prior to the valve click of aortic valve opening

origin and direction of the velocity jet may be unpredictable and careful transducer manipulation is required in order to confirm the presence of regurgitation in these patients. In addition, other transducer positions, within or outside the cardiac apex or an interspace higher, may be necessary to identify the systolic velocity jet and occasionally it will only be identified from the left parasternal edge. It should also be noted that the apical position which provides the best echocardiographic image is not always the exact position from which the best Doppler signal is obtained and the use of Doppler ultrasound with simultaneous imaging can, on occasions, provide a false sense of security.

Although simultaneous imaging can be helpful in the assessment of mitral prosthetic dysfunction, it is recommended that a dedicated continuous wave examination is performed in addition. By the use of this technique it is possible to identify a number of patients with minimal regurgitation and a very low intensity Doppler signal who would otherwise have been missed using only Doppler with simultaneous echocardiographic imaging. Painstaking examination from a variety of praecordial positions with careful manipulation of the Doppler beam and sample volume is of particular importance in patients with mechanical mitral replacements, since if the origin of the regurgitant jet is the result of a periprosthetic leak it will be detected with a different transducer position and angulation from which mitral diastolic flow is best identified.

The use of duplex scanners combining pulsed Doppler with simultaneous echocardiographic imaging allows the relationship of flow and structural detail and is valuable in identifying the origin of the regurgitant jet, whether it is due to a periprosthetic or through valve leak. Careful and meticulous examination around the valve prosthesis may be necessary to make this distinction, whereas the origin of the velocity jet will be more easily identified using real-time colour flow mapping (*see* Chapter 5). Even with careful examination from a variety of praecordial positions the possibility of missing a regurgitant mitral jet still exists, although this should rarely occur when regurgitation is significant.

If a non-imaging system is used, confusion can potentially occur between mitral regurgitation and severe aortic stenosis (*see* Chapter 4) and a similar problem exists with mitral prosthetic regurgitation. However, if the distinction is not apparent from the timing of the velocity signals they should be easily separated by the use of pulsed Doppler with simultaneous imaging. With mechanical prostheses the distinction is not difficult since the prominent valve clicks produced by the mechanical prosthesis make timing of any systolic flow velocity recording easy, and pansystolic mitral regurgitation will be readily separated from an ejection systolic aortic stenosis signal when using continuous wave Doppler.

Severity of mitral prosthetic regurgitation

Detection of the presence of mitral prosthetic regurgitation is a valuable clinical contribution of the technique but, clearly, this would be further enhanced if Doppler ultrasound could also provide some estimate as to its severity. The volume of blood travelling at a particular velocity and traversing the Doppler ultrasound beam will be related to the intensity of the spectral signal. Using continuous wave Doppler some assessment of the severity of regurgitation can be made from the signal intensity and although this is a very subjective method and can be affected by gain settings, it is of some value because it is relatively easy to perform. With pulsed Doppler, mapping of the extent of the regurgitant jet in the left atrium, as used in mitral valve disease[16, 17], can be applied to leaking valve prostheses[18]. Problems may arise with mechanical prostheses where poor ultrasound transmission through a pyrolitic carbon disc or steel ball may mask the presence of a regurgitant jet immediately behind the prosthesis. This would explain why regurgitation is not detected with normally functioning mechanical valves in the mitral position which, by their design, always have a minor degree of regurgitation. A further problem with this technique is the fact that pulsed Doppler will detect the presence of turbulent flow which may be distinct from the regurgitant jet and can falsely accentuate the severity of regurgitation, and failure to identify accurately the velocity jet will cause a false underestimation of its severity.

Despite these problems it is possible to provide some quantification of the severity of prosthetic regurgitation using this method. It is both difficult and time consuming to obtain meaningful results and requires meticulous examination by an experienced examiner. Patients with severe regurgitation will almost always be differentiated from those with only trivial regurgitation but, between these extremes, there is a large number where accurate quantification is impractical. The use of real-time colour flow mapping is in its infancy but its ability to provide a two-dimensional appreciation of Doppler flow velocity recordings with integration of structural detail has considerable potential both in detecting and assessing the severity of mitral prosthetic regurgitation. However, much work is required to determine the effect of haemodynamic variables on the spatial distribution of regurgitant jets with colour Doppler flow mapping.

Mitral diastolic flow velocity can also prove valuable in assessing the severity of regurgitation; severe regurgitation will produce an increase in diastolic forward flow velocity producing an increase in the maximum flow velocity without significant change in the mitral pressure half-time. Indeed, in the presence of regurgitation and a normal mitral pressure half-time, a peak mitral velocity across a bioprosthetic valve of greater than 2 m/s is highly suggestive of significant prosthetic regurgitation[5].

In practical terms in most cases the assessment of the severity of regurgitation is based on a combination of the above criteria and the expertise and experience of the operator, and although exact quantitation is not possible Doppler can provide additional valuable clinical information in a significant number of patients.

Aortic prosthetic regurgitation

Aortic prosthetic regurgitation should be sought in a similar way to aortic regurgitation in a native valve. The apical position should first be employed, the outflow tract imaged and the sample volume moved progressively through it to the valve. With a non-imaging transducer it is best studied initially with continuous wave Doppler by first locating mitral diastolic flow and then angling the transducer anteriorly and medially towards the aortic valve. If prosthetic aortic regurgitation is present it is almost always found by this technique, and is characterized by high velocity pandiastolic flow towards the transducer, usually of fairly low and uniform intensity (*Figure 9.9*). The signal itself is, not surprisingly, indistinguishable from that of aortic regurgitation related to aortic valve disease. Occasionally, the

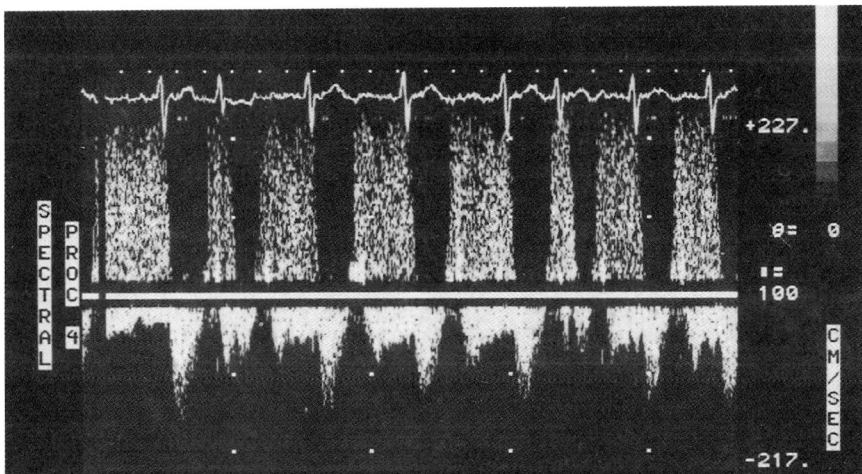

Figure 9.9 Continuous wave Doppler spectral display of aortic prosthetic regurgitation with low intensity high velocity signal seen throughout diastole

regurgitant jet is more easily found from the subcostal position but with aortic prostheses it is rarely found from the suprasternal or right parasternal positions. A semiquantitative assessment of the degree of regurgitation can be gained from the intensity of the continuous wave signal or the end diastolic velocity which indicates the diastolic pressure difference between the aorta and the left ventricle (*see* Chapter 4). A substantial fall in the flow velocity during diastole indicates a small end diastolic pressure difference and is characteristic of severe aortic prosthetic regurgitation (but will also be apparent from a high pulse pressure). Pulsed wave Doppler combined with simultaneous echo imaging can often distinguish between a para- and through-valve leak and may allow mapping of the extent of the velocity jet into the left ventricular cavity, providing some quantitation of the severity of regurgitation. This can usually identify those with only trivial regurgitation but, otherwise, its value is as yet unproven.

Aortic regurgitation *versus* obstructed mechanical mitral prosthesis

One potential problem with a non-imaging system is the separation of continuous wave Doppler recording of aortic regurgitation from a 'stuck' mitral disc valve in the same patient. In both cases the Doppler signal from the apical position will produce a high velocity diastolic signal towards the Doppler transducer, the stuck mitral prosthesis producing unusually high mitral diastolic velocities, similar in magnitude to those found in aortic regurgitation. The distinction will usually be obvious clinically, but a situation can arise in an extremely ill patient where confirmation of a severely obstructed mechanical mitral prosthesis may not be possible. Trivial aortic regurgitation may be undetected clinically and identification of this signal from the apex may give the false impression of an obstructed mitral disc valve. However, there is usually no difficulty in knowing the origin of the Doppler signal from the direction and position of the Doppler transducer and in patients with aortic regurgitation a separate, normal mitral prosthetic flow signal will be found. When mitral prosthetic clicks are identified then timing of the flow signal will additionally separate the two signals; aortic regurgitant flow will start before and mitral flow after opening of the mitral prosthesis. Furthermore, there tend to be higher intensity signals at the lower Doppler frequencies in patients with a stuck mechanical prosthesis, although this in itself is not sufficiently discriminating for critical clinical decisions to be based on it. It is noteworthy that the use of simultaneous echo imaging will not necessarily clarify any remaining doubts as to the origin of the signal since both can be found at a similar position within the left ventricular cavity. Colour Doppler flow mapping should allow this distinction to be made with certainty (*see Plate 16*).

Tricuspid regurgitation

Since tricuspid valve replacements are rare it is very unusual to encounter tricuspid prosthetic regurgitation, and its presence will usually be apparent clinically. Attempts at quantification by Doppler are probably of little clinical value, but the peak systolic velocity can be used to predict the pulmonary artery systolic pressure (*see* Chapter 6). Since attempts to cross a mechanical prosthesis at catheterization will not normally be undertaken, this can provide valuable information that may otherwise not be obtained.

Regurgitation of a native tricuspid valve is commonly identified by Doppler ultrasound even in normal individuals, and in patients with aortic and particularly mitral valve replacement, a tricuspid regurgitant signal can be demonstrated in as many as 90% of patients. It is therefore possible to predict the pulmonary artery systolic pressure non-invasively in a substantial proportion of these patients[19].

Clinical value of Doppler ultrasound

The potential clinical value of Doppler ultrasound in the assessment of prosthetic valve function is considerable. Clinical examination in these patients can often prove difficult, particularly where both mitral and aortic prostheses coexist and conventional non-invasive techniques can be unreliable. Although two-dimensional echocardiography can provide considerable structural detail it is a relatively insensitive technique for identifying prosthetic valve dysfunction and even less so for quantitating its severity. In particular, it is of little value in identifying the presence of mitral prosthetic regurgitation, which presents probably the most common clinical problem. Since an aortic valve prosthesis will usually produce a systolic murmur which may be widespread across the praecordium, the presence of regurgitation of a coexisting mitral valve replacement will often be questioned. Although the distinction may well be apparent clinically this is not always so, and the detection of mitral prosthetic regurgitation by Doppler ultrasound can provide clinically valuable information. If Doppler can provide some further assessment as to the severity of mitral prosthetic regurgitation it may, in certain patients, succeed where even invasive investigation has failed, as left ventricular angiography will not be possible when the aortic prosthesis is mechanical.

Similarly clinical assessment of the degree of obstruction of an aortic prosthesis is extremely difficult clinically, since all are, to a degree, obstructive even when functioning normally. Echocardiography can usually image the valve leaflets in a bioprosthesis but, as with aortic stenosis, the appearance of the valve may not always reflect the degree of obstruction. Measurement of the gradient across the aortic prosthesis will provide an accurate assessment of the degree of obstruction on which clinical judgements can be based, provided sufficient care is taken in performing the Doppler examination, and the potential problems of the technique or of missing a high velocity jet are borne in mind.

Thrombosis or obstruction from sticking of a mechanical mitral prosthesis is a rare but life-threatening situation which requires prompt surgical intervention. The diagnosis is usually suspected clinically, though confirmation is often sought prior to surgery and may involve a time consuming and hazardous catheterization procedure. The characteristic flow recording of an obstructed mechanical valve on continuous wave Doppler can provide rapid confirmation of the clinical problem and save valuable time in reaching corrective surgery.

Echocardiography often provides valuable structural detail of prosthetic valves but, because of the acoustic density of mechanical prostheses, rarely can it identify sufficient structural detail to suggest the presence of prosthetic valve dysfunction. Even with bioprosthetic valves echocardiography can be misleading. It can identify thickening or calcification of tissue leaflets where these can be well visualized, but it does not necessarily provide an accurate assessment of the degree of obstruction across the valve. In addition, the use of pericardial valves with improved haemodynamic properties has become more widespread and with some of the newer valve designs the development of leaflet tears or prolapse is the usual mode of valve failure. Somewhat surprisingly, echocardiography can easily miss these abnormalities, whereas Doppler ultrasound is extremely sensitive in identifying the presence of regurgitation through these prostheses, even when this is minor[6]. Follow-up of these patients by Doppler ultrasound may therefore identify a group of *at-risk* patients and optimize the timing of surgical intervention.

The major attraction of Doppler ultrasound is that it is non-invasive and easily repeatable, and it may prove valuable to perform an examination in all patients with valve replacements at regular intervals. Although this may be an ideal method of follow-up in centres where large numbers of valve replacements are performed each year, it will mean a substantial increase in the workload of the ultrasonographer and in certain centres it may be necessary to restrict repeated investigation to patients with suspected prosthetic valve dysfunction.

There are many continuing improvements in prosthetic valve design and, although much haemodynamic data can be accrued from studies *in vitro*, this does not always parallel the haemodynamic profile of a valve replacement *in vivo*. Adequate clinical data have only been possible previously either by measuring pressures across the valve at surgery, or by invasive catheterization procedures. Not only are these results obtained only at one point in time, either under the effects of sedation or anaesthesia but, in addition, they do not provide an adequate profile of prosthetic valve function under differing clinical situations. Doppler ultrasound can overcome these problems and provide a haemodynamic assessment of prosthetic valve function in patients under varying clincial situations over a period of time. Doppler ultrasound can therefore be of considerable clinical value and it also has a valuable research potential in the study of valve prostheses.

Doppler ultrasound can provide invaluable haemodynamic information on prosthetic valve function non-invasively. This technique should not be regarded in isolation, however, but, as with all Doppler assessment, as part of a complete clinical and non-invasive evaluation. It can provide information which would not otherwise be available to the clinician, and can obviate or direct the need for potentially hazardous invasive procedures in a significant number of these patients. The considerable clinical potential of the technique will be further advanced by the wider application of colour Doppler flow mapping (Chapter 11) which should enhance the substantial clinical impact that Doppler techniques already play in the patient with a prosthetic valve replacement.

References

1. ALAM, M., LAKIER, J. B., PICKARD, S. D. and GOLDSTEIN, S. (1983) Echocardiographic evaluation of porcine bioprosthetic valves: experience with 309 normal and 59 dysfunctioning valves. *Am. J. Cardiol.*, **52**, 309–315

2. BECKER, R. M., STROM, J., FRISHMAN, W. *et al*. (1980) Hemodynamic performance of the Ionescu-Shiley valve prosthesis. *J. Thorac. Cardiovasc. Surg.*, **80**, 613–620

3. COSGROVE, D. M., LYTLE, B. W., GILL, C. C. *et al*. (1985) *In vivo* hemodynamic comparison of porcine and pericardial valves. *J. Thorac. Cardiovasc. Surg.*, **89**, 358–368

4. WILLIAMS, G. A. and LABOVITZ, A. J. (1985) Doppler hemodynamic evaluation of prosthetic (Starr–Edwards and Bjork–Shiley) and bioprosthetic (Hancock and Carpentier–Edwards) cardiac valves. *Am. J. Cardiol.*, **56**, 325–332

5. RYAN, T., ARMSTRONG, W. F., DILLON, J. C. and FEIGENBAUM, H. (1986) Doppler echocardiographic evaluation of patients with porcine mitral valves. *Am. Heart J.*, **111**, 237–244

6. SIMPSON, I. A., REECE, I. J., HOUSTON, A. B., HUTTON, I., WHEATLEY, D. J. and COBBE, S. M. (1986) Non-invasive haemodynamic assessment of 155 patients with bioprosthetic valves by Doppler ultrasound: a comparison of the Wessex porcine, low profile Ionescu Shiley and Hancock pericardial bioprostheses. *Br. Heart J.*, **56**, 83–88

7. SIMPSON, I. A., FISHER, J., REECE, I. J., HOUSTON, A. B., HUTTON, I. and WHEATLEY, D. J. (1986) Comparison of Doppler ultrasound velocity measurements with pressure differences across bioprosthetic valves in a pulsatile flow model. *Cardivasc. Res.*, **20**, 317–321

8. WEINSTEIN, I. R., MARBARGER, J. P. and PEREZ, J. E. (1983) Ultrasonic assessment of the St Jude prosthetic valve: M-mode, two dimensional and Doppler echocardiography. *Circulation*, **68**, 897–905

9. HOLEN, J., SIMONSEN, S. and FROYSAKER, T. (1981) Determination of pressure gradient in the Hancock mitral valve from noninvasive Doppler data. *Scand. J. Clin. Lab. Invest.*, **41**, 177–183

10. HOLEN, J., SIMONSEN, S. and FROYSAKER, T. (1979) An ultrasound Doppler technique for the noninvasive determination of the pressure gradient in the Bjork–Shiley mitral valve. *Circulation*, **59**, 436–442

11. SIMPSON, I. A., HOUSTON, A. B., RODGER, J. C., TWEDDEL, A. C. and HUTTON, I. (1986) Haemodynamic assessment of mitral valve prostheses by non-invasive Doppler ultrasound. *J. Cardiovas. Ultrasonography*, **5**, 353–358

12. WALKER, D. K., SCOTTEN, L. N., MODI, V. J. and BROWNLEE, R. T. (1980) *In vitro* assessment of mitral valve prostheses. *J. Thorac. Cardiovasc. Surg*, **79**, 680–688

13. YOGANATHAN, A. P., WOO, Y. R., WILLIAMS, F. P., STEVENSON, D. M., FRANCH, R. H. and HARRISON, E. C. (1983) *In vitro* fluid dynamic characteristics of Ionescu–Shiley and Carpentier Edwards tissue bioprostheses. *Artificial Organs*, **7**, 459–469

14. MANN, D. L., GILLAM, L. D., MARSHALL, J. E., KING, M. E. and WEYMAN, A. E. (1986) Doppler and two-dimensional echocardiographic diagnosis of Bjork–Shiley prosthetic valve malfunction: importance of interventricular septal motion and timing of onset of valve flow. *J. Am. Coll. Cardiol.*, **8**, 971–974

15. WILKES, H. S., BERGER, M., GALLERSTEIN, P. E., BERDOFF, R. L. and GOLDBERG, E. (1983) Left ventricular outflow obstruction after aortic valve replacement: detection with continuous wave Doppler ultrasound recording. *J. Am. Coll. Cardiol.*, **1**, 550–553

16. MIYATAKE, K., KINOSHITA, N., NAGATA, S. *et al.* (1980) Intracardiac flow patterns in mitral regurgitation studied with combined use of the ultrasonic pulsed Doppler technique and cross-sectional echocardiography. *Am. J. Cardiol.*, **45**, 155–162

17. QUINONES, M. A., YOUNG, J. B., WAGGONER, A. D., OSTOJIC, M. C., RIBEIRO, L. G. T. and MILLER, R. R. (1980) Assessment of pulsed Doppler echocardiography in detection and quantification of aortic and mitral regurgitation. *Br. Heart J.*, **44**, 612–620

18. VEYRAT, C., WITCHITZ, S., LESSANA, A., AMEUR, A., ABITBOL, G. and KALMANSON, D. (1985) Valvar prosthetic dysfunction: localisation and evaluation of the dysfunction using the Doppler technique. *Br. Heart J.*, **54**, 273–284

19. BERGER, M., HAIMOWITZ, A., VAN TOSH, A., BERDOFF, R. L. and GOLDBERG, E. (1985) Quantitative assessment of pulmonary hypertension in patients with tricuspid regurgitation using continuous wave Doppler ultrasound. *J. Am. Coll. Cardiol.*, **6**, 359–365

10

Measurement of cardiac output

Terje Skjaerpe

The assessment of cardiac output plays an important role in the management of patients who are critically ill, particularly following acute myocardial infarction, or who have chronic congestive cardiac failure. As a result the measurement of cardiac output by the thermodilution technique using a Swan–Ganz catheter has become a valuable and established procedure. Because of its invasive nature this technique is not entirely free from risk and, because of potential complications, can only be utilized for a few days at a time. An easily repeatable, non-invasive method of accurately measuring cardiac output would have considerable advantages, not only in critically ill patients requiring careful haemodynamic monitoring, but also in relatively healthy patients or volunteer subjects taking part in clinical trials, where the small but definite risk of right heart catheterization is unacceptable. Doppler ultrasound can measure flow velocity and, if the cross-sectional area of the vessel can be measured by echocardiography, then theoretically, multiplication of the flow velocity by the area should provide a non-invasive estimation of cardiac output. Although this formula is simple in theory, there are many potential problems associated with its application.

The assessment of cardiac output by a combination of Doppler ultrasound and echocardiography has been the subject of extensive research. When the literature is reviewed it becomes apparent that no general agreement has been reached on how the measurement of either the flow velocity or area should be made, even when only the outflow system from the left ventricle is considered[1–5]. It is therefore not possible to be dogmatic about the most appropriate technique for the measurement of cardiac output.

Most of the present author's experience, and the major part of experimental and clinical studies, have been on volumetric flow estimation in the left ventricular outflow tract and ascending aorta. This chapter thus concentrates on the technique and problems relating to the use of this site, but since many of these also apply to others, their advantages and disadvantages will also be considered.

Volumetric flow estimation in the aorta and its outflow tract

Theoretical considerations

Volumetric flow

The theoretical basis for calculating volumetric flow by Doppler echocardiography is that the flow velocity (cm/s) is multiplied by the area (cm^2) across which flow occurs to provide an estimate of volumetric flow (ml/s). This is then multiplied by 60 (to give ml/minute) and divided by 1000 to give cardiac output (CO) in l/minute.

$$\text{Thus: cardiac output (l/min)} = \frac{\text{area(cm}^2) \times \text{velocity (cm/s)} \times 60}{1000} \text{ (see appendix)}$$

The velocity used to assess cardiac output should be neither the peak nor the mean systolic velocity from a given spectral signal but the average velocity occurring over the whole cardiac cycle, known as the *time averaged velocity* (*see* Chapter 1). A range of velocities are demonstrated on the spectrum analyser and these vary throughout the cardiac cycle; at any point in time both the maximum and instantaneous velocity can be measured. The curve plotting the change of these with time can be drawn. By measuring the area under (or integrating) the velocity signal curve, either electronically or by planimetry, and dividing it by the duration of the cycle the average velocity throughout the cardiac cycle, known as the *time averaged mean* or *time averaged maximum velocity* is obtained. Each of these measurements will depend on the velocity profile of flow within the vessel studied.

For estimation of cardiac output the velocity should also be averaged across the whole of the flow area to produce the *spatial* or *space averaged velocity* as opposed to that obtained from only a small part of the flow area. Since the ultrasound sample volume commonly used with pulsed Doppler is much smaller than the cross-sectional flow area the accuracy of Doppler measurement used in the calculation thereafter depends on the degree to which this represents the mean spatial velocity across the whole vessel. The space averaged velocity would be obtained if the width of the Doppler sample beam encompassed the whole of the orifice area and all the velocities across the vessel area could then be measured. If the velocity profile across the flow area is flat, i.e. the blood is moving at the same velocity across the whole of the orifice area, then the velocities identified in the region of a relatively small Doppler beam will be representative of the space averaged velocity. However, if the velocity profile is not flat, but parabolic, then sampling from a region near the centre of the vessel, where the velocities would be higher than near the vessel wall, would tend to overestimate the space averaged velocity. Similarly, if the velocity profile is skewed, i.e. higher velocities are present at one side of the vessel than the other, and the Doppler sample beam is directed at the higher or lower velocities, overestimation or underestimation of the space averaged velocity, and hence the cardiac output, will occur.

The assumption of a flat velocity profile in the ascending aorta in humans is based on experimental studies, mostly on dogs, where a fairly flat, although to some extent skewed, velocity profile is found[6]. On the other hand, studies in horses[7] recorded significantly higher velocities in the proximal than distal part of the ascending aorta, despite a larger diameter at the proximal level; this finding is incompatible with a flat velocity profile in the aortic root. One should therefore be careful in applying results obtained in animal studies to humans.

The skewed velocity profile found in dogs is in accordance with flow theory[6]. This suggests that in a curved flow channel, higher velocities are found at the inner curvature in the first part of the bend while downstream redistribution of flow velocities occurs with higher velocities at the outer curvature. Other experimental studies have found the central velocity to be close to the spatial mean[6] and found the effect of temporal skewing to be of little importance when the velocities were integrated during the whole of systole[8].

The existence of a skewed velocity profile in the ascending aorta has also been demonstrated in man[9], and in contrast to the experimental study[8] a variation in the time–velocity integral was observed depending upon the position of the sample volume.

The theoretical basis for a flat velocity profile is that the aorta constitutes a narrow flow channel of constant diameter branching off a larger one, the left ventricle. In this situation a flat velocity profile is to be expected at the inlet to the narrower channel. However, measurement of the diameter at different levels in the ascending aorta[10], has shown that it is not of constant diameter and considerable dilatation of the ascending aorta often occurs; even at its narrowest level, the sinotubular junction, the cross-sectional area can be up to 200% larger than the area at the annulus. This dilatation of the ascending aorta, compared with the annulus, increases with age. Thus, in contrast to the theoretical model, blood is often ejected through a narrow annulus into a wide aorta where the flow pattern will probably be similar to that distal to an obstruction. This means that during the acceleration phase, the narrow core of flow at the annulus expands to give a fairly flat profile at a short distance downstream and a spectral display will show a narrow frequency band on the upstroke part of the curve (*Figure 10.1*). At the sides of the expanding core of flow, eddies are formed and during the deceleration phase these expand downstream. Because of the curved course of the aorta, the eddies will be largest at the inner curvature and spectral broadening will be observed possibly with a rapid decrease of velocities and a tendency to negative velocities at end systole. At the outer curvature the forward flowing component of the eddies may result in forward velocities being recorded even after aortic valve closure (*Figure 10.1*). The resulting deformation of the velocity profile makes it difficult to define a position where velocities representing the spatial mean can be recorded. If the

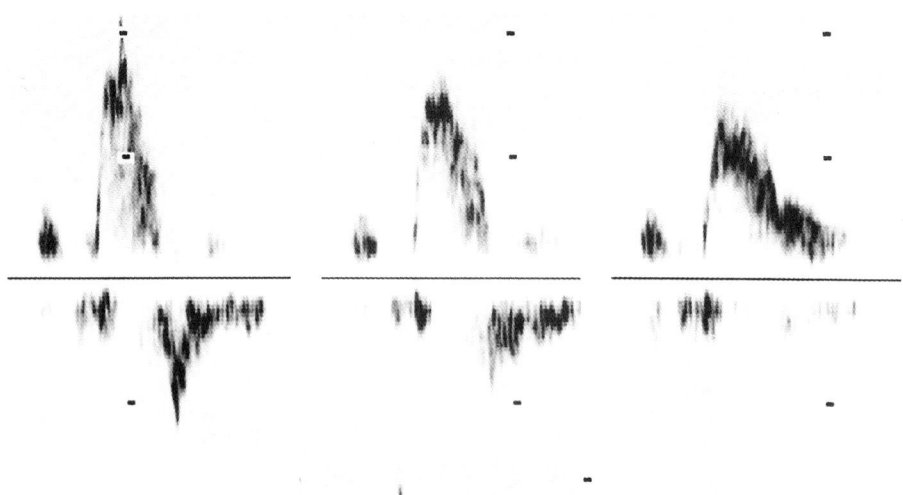

Figure 10.1 Doppler recordings in the ascending aorta from a single individual obtained at the inner curvature (left), the centre (middle), and outer curvature (right). Probably because of a large eddy developing in late systole, negative velocities are recorded at the inner bend before aortic valve closure while positive velocities are recorded at the outer bend. Spectral broadening of the deceleration part of the curve is also shown

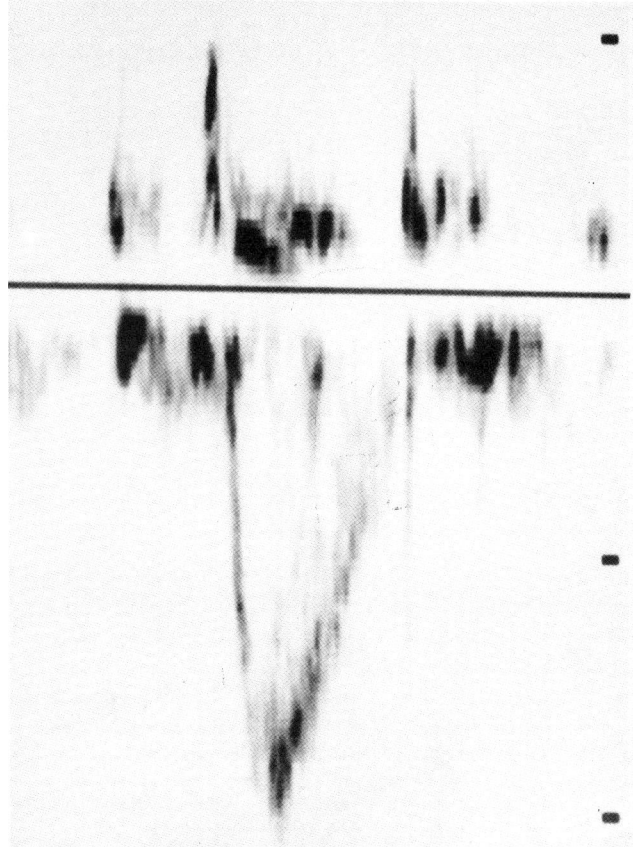

Figure 10.2 Recording in the immediate subvalve area. There is less spectral broadening and minimal tendency to positive or negative velocities at end systole

highest velocities obtained are used in the calculation of cardiac output it is likely to be overestimated. The progressive dilatation of the aorta with age means that a more complex velocity pattern is to be expected in adults or older patients than in children and the problems of accurately measuring mean velocity will be greater.

In the subvalve area there is a decrease in cross-sectional flow area from the left ventricle to the annulus. The blood is therefore subjected to convective acceleration, even at the end of systole, stabilizing and flattening the velocity profile and preventing the formation of eddies. This phenomenon is reflected in the spectral velocity recordings by the limited spectral broadening of both the upstroke and downstroke part of the velocity curve (*Figure 10.2*). No unexpected positive or negative velocities are recorded at end systole.

Diameter measurements

If Doppler ultrasound is to provide an accurate assessment of volumetric cardiac output, it is not enough to be able to measure flow velocity; an accurate assessment of the cross-sectional area over which flow is occurring is essential. Echocardio-graphy is the only practical choice as a non-invasive method of measuring the aortic cross-sectional area, but there are a number of potential problems and it is essential to know of them. The aorta is a dynamic structure with expansion of the flow area during systole and with increasing cardiac output. The size of the outflow tract varies from the subvalve area, to the annulus, and ascending aorta. In addition, the area will vary depending on whether it is measured from a two-dimensional image by planimetry or calculated from the radius measured from an M-mode or two-dimensional record as leading to leading or trailing to leading edge.

Conventionally echocardiographic measurements are made as leading to leading edge and this will give the most accurate assessment of size. However, when combining this measurement with Doppler measurement of velocity there may be reasons for not adhering to this convention. If diameter measurements are taken from the ascending aorta these should be made as trailing to leading edge at the sinotubular junction which marks the narrowest part of the ascending aorta distal to the annulus. This may to some extent compensate for the tendency towards overestimation of the spatial mean velocity occurring when the profile is not flat and the highest velocities which can be obtained with Doppler are used for this calculation.

At the level of the aortic annulus, just below the insertion of the aortic valve leaflets, the situation is different because of a flatter velocity profile. Although in theory the leading to leading edge diameter measurements may be more correct at this level[4], the leading edge of the anterior echo can be difficult to define in some patients. In addition, friction between the endocardium and the blood produces a narrow zone with lower velocities (the boundary layer) close to the walls. The effective flow area is thus slightly narrower than the anatomical area. The use of trailing to leading edge measurements is thus justified provided that gain is adjusted carefully to avoid excessively strong echoes which would further reduce the measured diameter.

The measurement should be made using two-dimensional echocardiography to ensure a beam direction from which the anterior and posterior parts of the annulus can best be recorded simultaneously to provide the most accurate measurement of the anteroposterior diameter. To utilize the advantage of high axial resolution a parasternal transducer position is preferred to an apical or suprasternal one. The flow area is generally assumed to be circular so that it can be calculated from the measurement of the radius (πr^2). This may not always be true, and theoretically it should be visualized in the short axis plane and the area measured by planimetry. However, since the annulus exhibits considerable axial movements during the cardiac cycle and part of the circumference is subjected to the poor lateral resolution of two-dimensional echocardiographic instruments, it is more appropri-ate to use the much simpler diameter measurement procedure in the majority of cases.

Results from a study on open chest dogs[11] suggested that measurement of flow area should be repeated when changes in flow rate were recorded. However, no significant difference has been found in the aortic orifice area between diastole and systole[4] and it seems sufficient to measure the area once during any series of cardiac output measurements. Thus changes in flow rate should be mirrored by changes in the velocity integral, which suggests that the use of Doppler ultrasound to reflect changes in cardiac output in an individual subject remains valid.

Doppler recordings

The foregoing sections have indicated that there is no universally agreed site and means of making either the Doppler or dimension measurement. In principle, there are two ways in which the Doppler measurements can be made: the highest velocities can be recorded either by continuous wave Doppler or by careful scanning in pulsed mode, or the velocities can be recorded with pulsed Doppler at a defined site. In some studies, the highest velocities combined with the diameter at the sinotubular junction have produced good estimates of cardiac output[2], while in others cardiac output was considerably overestimated in some patients when the highest velocities were combined with any diameter distal to the annulus[4]. The largest overestimation occurred in those with the greatest dilatation of the ascending aorta compared with the annulus, and the apparently conflicting results may be explained by different patient groups. Therefore, in a completely unselected patient group caution should be exercised when using the highest velocity in the ascending aorta together with any measurement of diameter distal to the annulus.

No studies have yet shown that it is possible to select specific levels for both velocity and diameter measurements in the ascending aorta in patients with the aorta dilated distal to the annulus. On the other hand, if the ascending aorta is found to be of even calibre by two-dimensional echocardiography, and similar to that at the annulus, the velocity profile is probably quite flat, allowing such measurements to be made. Because of the skewing of the velocity profile, central recordings should be made. This is best carried out with an imaging transducer but, by scanning from side to side with a non-imaging one, the selection of the velocity representing the cross-sectional mean can be made fairly reliably.

In a few patients it is possible to underestimate cardiac output by recording the highest velocities from the suprasternal notch and the diameter at the annulus. In these patients higher velocities will be recorded from the right parasternal border because the axis of the aortic root is more horizontal than usual; the angle between the direction of flow and the ultrasound beam directed from the suprasternal notch is greater than usual and, if no allowance is made for the angle of incidence of the Doppler beam to blood flow, there will be subsequent underestimation of flow velocity.

Although velocity recordings from the suprasternal notch can be obtained in most patients, velocities in the subvalve area and aorta can also be obtained from the apical position. Theoretically several problems should be eliminated when the velocities are recorded in the immediate subvalve area from the apex. In particular, the assumption of a flat velocity profile will be valid and the transducer position can be more easily adjusted to reduce the angle of incidence of the Doppler beam with flow. In addition, an imaging transducer is more easily used from this position.

If poor acoustic windows limit the number of possible recording positions, one should be aware that, from the apical position the angle can become sufficiently large to produce significant underestimation of velocity and cardiac output. Under these circumstances it is prudent to record the velocity in the aortic root from the right parasternal border and the suprasternal notch. If significantly higher velocities can be recorded from these positions then underestimation of the velocity from the apex must be suspected, providing aortic stenosis has been excluded as a cause of the increased velocity. This can be carried out by Doppler by moving the sample volume out of the left ventricular outflow tract and through the aortic valve, excluding any stepwise increase in velocity.

In clinical practice an important practical advantage of measuring the velocity below the aortic valve is that it seems possible to obtain a useful estimation of cardiac output in patients with aortic stenosis, providing a basis for non-invasive assessment of the valve area as discussed in Chapter 4. Furthermore, in the presence of associated aortic regurgitation, the total stroke volume will be estimated, making assessment of valve area independent of the effect of the regurgitation.

Estimation of volumetric flow at other sites

Pulmonary artery

In principle, the problems of estimating cardiac output in the ascending aorta apply equally to the pulmonary artery. In practice, however, its lateral wall often cannot be visualized clearly, making measurement of its diameter impossible. Therefore most clinical studies of pulmonary flow have been performed on children in whom satisfactory echocardiographic images of the pulmonary artery are more readily obtained. This is precisely the age group in which intracardiac shunts present clinical problems and assessment of both left- and right-sided cardiac output becomes important for the calculation of pulmonary/systemic flow ratios (QP/QS). Although the potential problem of dilatation of the pulmonary artery relative to the annulus with increasing age is of little importance, dilatation caused by increased flow from intracardiac shunts may present problems. Little experimental evidence exists on its effect upon the velocity profile. However, clinical studies have reported accurate estimation of pulmonary flow in such patients[12, 13], possibly because the annulus also dilates to some extent, reducing the variation in calibre. However, in some patients with pulmonary hypertension and dilatation of the pulmonary artery, different velocity curves have been recorded when the sample volume is moved from one side of the artery to the other. If this occurs it is probably wise to measure the diameter and velocity only at the level of the annulus.

The course of the pulmonary artery is such that diameter measurements suffer from the poor lateral resolution of two-dimensional echocardiography and, particularly in small children, this may give rise to significant errors. For example, if the diameter of the vessel is 10 mm, an error of 1 mm in the diameter measurement produces an error of about 20% in estimated cardiac output, while in a vessel with a diameter of 20 mm, an error of 1 mm causes a 10% error.

Mitral and tricuspid valves

The measurement of flow area at the atrioventricular valves presents different problems from those experienced in the aorta and the pulmonary artery. The mitral annulus is an ellipse of variable shape which becomes more circular at end diastole. Area changes of about 14% during diastole, and 26% throughout the cardiac cycle have been reported[14]. Unlike the left ventricular outlet, a significant increase in the area can occur with increasing flow rate[11] and it is important to be aware of the possible need for repeated measurements of flow area with changes in flow rate.

The flow area at the level of the mitral valve leaflets exhibits even larger variations than at the annulus. The area is generally assumed to be elliptical with a constant large diameter and a variable small one. The area between the leaflets on an M-mode echocardiogram is integrated and divided by the diastolic flow time to provide an estimate of a mean small axis diameter. This is then divided by the maximal leaflet separation and multiplied by the maximal mitral valve opening as measured with two-dimensional echocardiography to give a corrected mitral valve area. This is then used together with the integral of velocity recordings at the tip of the mitral valve to calculate cardiac output[15, 16]. Since the mathematically correct procedure would be to integrate the instantaneous product of flow velocity and flow area over time, the simplified method commonly used introduces further errors in calculation in addition to those in measurement.

The velocity profile at the level of the mitral valve annulus is flat but at the level of the leaflets a skew is observed in mid- and late diastole, and it is likely that a tendency to overestimate the flow rate will result from the use of the highest velocities recorded.

Practical application of the technique

Theoretical and clinical evidence both indicate that the aortic annulus is the optimal level at which to make diameter and velocity measurements for calculation of cardiac output. For echocardiographic study it has the advantages that axial imaging planes can be used to measure the diameter, a circular shape can be assumed, the area remains constant with variation in flow, and its proximity to the chest wall makes it easier to visualize in patients in whom it is difficult to obtain satisfactory echocardiographic images of deeper structures. Furthermore, for the Doppler study a flat velocity profile is more likely at this than at any other level in the heart or the great vessels. Nevertheless, quite acceptable estimates of cardiac output can be obtained by using other positions in the ascending aorta in children and certain other groups of patients.

The velocity measurements are best made using pulsed Doppler with the transducer in an apical site and the patient in the left lateral position. Although an imaging transducer may simplify the procedure its use is not necessary, and in patients in whom it is difficult to obtain a good Doppler signal the higher sensitivity of a separate Doppler transducer is a definite advantage and more important than the image in obtaining the best velocity recording.

The optimal position for the sample volume is obtained by moving it out through the left ventricular outflow tract until the closure sound of the aortic valve is heard as a distinct click in the audio signal and recorded on the spectral display. The procedure should be repeated from positions medial and lateral to the apex to ensure that the highest velocities are recorded. As part of the procedure aortic stenosis should be excluded by moving the sample volume through the aortic valve as previously described.

The motion of the mitral valve and perhaps the septum, may produce strong, low frequency diastolic signals which may be included in the tracing by an automatic integrator with resultant overestimating of the flow rate. A higher setting of the high pass filter may solve this problem, but since it shortens the ejection time as determined by the computer, the velocity integral is reduced. Small adjustments of the sample volume position may improve the signal while manual tracing of the spectral curves eliminates it completely. In sinus rhythm beats during the whole of at least one respiratory cycle should be averaged, while in atrial fibrillation at least 10 beats should be included.

In patients with a mitral valve prosthesis or subvalvar obstruction the anatomy of the left ventricular outflow tract, and consequently the velocity pattern, is disturbed. Caution should then be exerted in estimating volume flow at this level. Similarly a ventricular septal defect in the upper part of the septum may present problems in obtaining satisfactory and reliable recordings.

Even at an optimal level, the reproducibility of ultrasound measurements presents limits on the accuracy of the non-invasive method. With echocardiography inaccuracies in diameter measurements up to 2 mm are to be expected in some adult patients and, depending on the size of the left ventricular outflow tract, errors of 15–20% in cardiac output will result. The smallest detectable change in velocity seems to be about 10%[17]. The combined error can then be up to 25–30%, although in practice it is probably less. If a maximal velocity estimator is used, or if the envelope of a spectral curve is traced, the flow rate will be slightly over-estimated when the velocity profile is not completely flat. On the other hand, one of the most important errors in measuring the diameter is probably that the imaging plane may not be at the midpoint of the vessel. The diameter and consequently the area is then underestimated, partly compensating for any overestimation made by the Doppler velocity recordings. When the invasive methods can themselves produce an error of up to 20%[18], the excellent correlation often reported between Doppler and invasive measurements of cardiac output may seem somewhat surprising. However, it should always be remembered that although the correlation coefficient is high, the absolute deviation between the two methods has been up to 40% in some studies. This is as might well be expected when the potential errors of both the invasive and non-invasive methods are combined. Thus care must be exercised in applying any individual result to clinical practice.

The availability of other measurement sites is important in that volume fractions (regurgitant and shunt volumes), or the effective cardiac output in case of aortic regurgitation, can be estimated. Since errors up to 25% may occur from measurements made in the left ventricular outflow tract, which is the most suitable site for volumetric flow measurements, the errors are likely to be even larger at other sites. Caution should therefore be exercised in drawing conclusions when volumetric flow at two different sites is compared with quantitative volume fractions. More research is needed to evaluate the extent to which measurement errors at the various sites are comparable within an individual; if they are not significant errors in estimation of shunts and regurgitant fractions may result.

Since there is considerable variation in equipment, expertise, patient population, etc., and the present author has limited experience of other sites, a dogmatic opinion cannot be given and the reader might consider it appropriate to judge from the literature which method is likely to work best in his own laboratory rather than simply following these recommendations. Whenever possible validation of the technique within an indivdual laboratory is recommended to ensure the correct interpretation of the results prior to clinical application of the method.

Experience in children seems to indicate that measurement at the pulmonary artery site provides a useful estimation of right ventricular output when flow is not disturbed by a shunt through a ventricular septal defect. Recording at the level of the annulus is theoretically best. If, in a given patient, it appears easier to measure flow and diameter distal to the annulus, the cross-section of the artery should be scanned with the sample volume; in the event of an uneven velocity distribution, velocity curves at different positions should be integrated and averaged. For serial measurements, the position giving the velocity curve closest to the cross-sectional mean should be chosen.

Published reports give no clear recommendation on which procedure should be used to measure flow through the mitral valve. Since the velocity profile is flattest at the annulus, it is most appropriate to make the measurements at this level and as the shape of the annulus is elliptical rather than circular, to measure two diameters and calculate the area by the formula of elliptical areas. However, the mitral annulus exhibits considerable axial movement during diastole, altering the position of the Doppler sample volume relative to it and careful positioning of the sample volume with an imaging transducer is therefore essential. Since the flow area will decrease from the annulus to the tips of the mitral leaflets during part of the diastole, there is also a change in the velocity curve such that Doppler recordings are most easily made at the level of the leaflets where the smallest flow area and thus the highest velocities occur during most of diastole. The use of this site is impractical for routine purposes since measurement of flow area is quite laborious. However, should it be chosen, the inner border of the leaflets should be used to digitize the maximal valve opening on two-dimensional echocardiographic recordings to avoid significant overestimation of cardiac output caused by the fact that the velocity profile is not completely flat at this level.

The theoretical difficulties in measuring cardiac output at the mitral valve site have been confirmed by the mixed clinical experience. The interobserver variability in cardiac output estimations at the mitral annulus level is also reported to be higher ($16.4\% \pm 13.8\%$) than at aortic annulus level ($6.8\% \pm 5.11\%$)[3]. The accuracy of cardiac output measurements at the mitral valve site thus needs further evaluation, and at present the method cannot be recommended for use in routine clinical practice.

There is little clinical experience on the estimation of cardiac output through the tricuspid valve. The problems relating to the mitral valve are similar to those with the tricuspid valve; although the annulus may be more circular, making area measurements simpler, the lower velocities at this level may reduce the accuracy of velocity integration. Thus further evaluation is required and considerable doubt must remain as to the potential value of this site for cardiac output estimation.

Clinical application

Estimation of cardiac output from the aorta with Doppler provides a fairly accurate comparison with invasive methods. Until now invasive techniques have been the only practical means of measuring cardiac output and although they have become regarded as the 'gold standard' it must be remembered that there are a number of problems associated with their application. Indeed, under highly controlled conditions *in vitro* significant systematic errors of thermodilution compared with pump output have been found with deviation between them of up to 23.5%[18]. The Fick principle is reasonably accurate in low cardiac output situations where the arteriovenous oxygen difference is large. In high output states, however, the narrow oxygen gap allows only rough estimates of cardiac output[19]. In addition it can be fairly complicated, increasing the risk of errors being made.

It is necessary to consider the criteria by which patients should be selected for invasive or non-invasive measurements of cardiac output. The prime requirement for the non-invasive ultrasonic method is that the acoustic conditions allow echocardiographic and Doppler measurements to be made with acceptable accuracy. Since this requires that the patient be turned on his side when necessary, the postoperative patient is not ideal, especially if he has undergone cardiac or thoracic surgery when it becomes difficult to use the optimal chest positions or obtain satisfactory recordings. In these patients monitoring of cardiac output is needed for only a few days and thermodilution becomes the obvious choice although, in children, the volume of fluid used may preclude repeated measurements. Recent experience would indicate that significant advantages can be gained in comparison with thermodilution by the use of a Doppler ultrasound probe attached to the aorta at the end of the operation. Since the aortic diameter can be measured accurately at surgery it is possible to monitor cardiac output continuously for several days[20], after which the transducer is removed through the chest drain and resterilized for subsequent use.

In patients in whom a right heart catheterization is considered necessary for other reasons, Fick or thermodilution remains the natural choice.

In the coronary care unit the advantages and disadvantages of each method are less clear. There are small but significant risks associated with right heart catheterization and the insertion of a Swan–Ganz catheter is probably more worrying to the patient than an ultrasound examination. Thus, if only one or two cardiac output measurements are considered necessary, Doppler may be the most appropriate choice but, in critically ill patients, where repeated measurements are necessary, thermodilution may be less disturbing than a series of Doppler recordings.

Clearly, Doppler is the ideal method when cardiac output measurements are part of the evaluation of outpatients. In the patient with aortic stenosis and both aortic and mitral regurgitation, Doppler estimates of aortic flow rates provide the only methods to estimate the valve area.

It is hoped that this chapter has demonstrated that one of the major problems associated with the non-invasive assessment of cardiac output by Doppler ultrasound is the difficulty in accurately estimating the flow area, with any error being increased when the radius is squared to obtain the cross-sectional area. Since the flow area at the aortic annulus does not seem to change within an individual patient or with varying flow rates, diameter measurements will not influence the changes observed in Doppler estimation of cardiac output at this site thus reducing errors in estimation to about 10%. Doppler ultrasound may therefore prove an ideal method for assessing relative changes in cardiac output within an individual. Since it allows measurements to be made under more physiological conditions than those of the catheterization laboratory and makes serial measurements easier, it is likely to prove superior to other methods of cardiac output assessment in patients in whom it is important to evaluate the effect of therapy[21]. It may have particular clinical value in the assessment of the haemodynamic response to varying pacemaker modalities by allowing relative changes in cardiac output to be assessed rapidly, thus serving as a guide to both the type of pacemaker inserted and the optimal pacing modality[22]. In these patients a considerable number of cardiac output estimations can be performed in a short space of time as pacemaker settings are adjusted. Similar estimations using thermodilution techniques would necessitate large quantities of fluid, potentially up to 1.5 litres, with possible deleterious effects in patients with compromised ventricular function.

Conclusions

It is necessary to accept some limitations on the accuracy of Doppler in the estimation of absolute flow volume which is necessary in certain clinical situations. However, there is good reason to believe that the accuracy of the most commonly used invasive methods, Fick and thermodilution, is only moderately higher. Certainly, Doppler demands more cooperation from the patient than thermodilution, but less than is required by the Fick method. The major advantage of the Doppler technique is that it is completely non-invasive, and can provide an accurate reflection of changes in cardiac output, often as important as absolute values. The use of the aortic annulus for velocity and diameter measurements is likely to prove the most accurate, but will not give an exact comparison with thermodilution. Although there are problems in the Doppler estimation of cardiac output, if the technique is applied with full knowledge of these limitations, it represents a valuable adjunct to other methods of assessing this and in some situations may prove the method of choice.

References

1. LOEPPKY, J. A., HOEKENGA, D. E., GREENE, E. R. and LUFT, U. C. (1984) Comparison of non-invasive pulsed Doppler and Fick measurements of stroke volume in cardiac patients. *Am. Heart J.*, **107**, 339–346

2. HUNTSMAN, L. L., STEWART, D. K., BARNES, S. R., FRANKLIN, S. B., COLOCOUSIS, J. S. and HESSEL, E. A. (1983) Non-invasive Doppler determination of cardiac output in man. Clinical validation. *Circulation*, **67**, 593–602

3. LEWIS, J. F., KUO, L. C., NELSON, J. G., LIMACHER, M. C. and QUINONES, M. A. (1984) Pulsed Doppler echocardiographic determination of stroke volume and cardiac output. Clinical validation of two new methods using the apical window. *Circulation*, **70**, 425–431

4. IHLEN, H., AMLIE, J. P., DALE, J. *et al.* (1984) Determination of cardiac output by Doppler echocardiography. *Br. Heart J.*, **51**, 54–60

5. LABOVITZ, A. J., BUCKINGHAM, T. A., HABERMEHL, K., NELSON, J. KENNEDY, H. L. and WILLIAMS, G. A. (1985) The effect of the sampling site on the two-dimensional echo Doppler determination of cardiac output. *Am. Heart J.*, **109**, 327–332

6. SEED, W. A. and WOOD, N. B. (1971) Velocity patterns in the aorta. *Cardiovasc. Res.*, **5**, 319–330

7. NEREM, R. M., RUMBERGER, J. A., GROSS, D. R., HAMLIN, R. L. and GEIGER, G. L. (1974) Hot-film anemometer velocity measurements of arterial blood flow in horses. *Circulation Res.*, **XXXIV**, 193–203

8. FISHER, D. C., SAHN, D. J., FRIEDMAN, M. J. *et al.* (1983) The effect of variations on pulsed Doppler sampling site on calculation of cardiac output: an experimental study in open-chest dogs. *Circulation*, **67**, 370–376

9. JENNI, R., VIELI, A., RUFFMAN, K., KRAYENBUEHL, H. P. and ANLIKER, M. (1984) A comparison between single gate and multigate Doppler measurements for the assessment of the velocity pattern in the human ascending aorta. *Eur. Heart J.*, **5**, 948–953

10. SKJAERPE, T. (1986) Influence of the geometry of the ascending aorta upon the velocity profile. In *Cardiac Doppler Diagnosis*, Vol. II, edited by M. P. Spencer, pp. 65–71. Boston: Martinus Nijhoff Publishers

11. STEWART, W. J., JIANG, L., MICH, R., PANDIAN, N., GUERRERO, J. L. and WEYMAN, A. E. (1985) Variable effects of changes in flow rate through the aortic, pulmonary, and mitral valves on valve area and flow velocity. Impact on quantitative Doppler flow calculations. *J. Am. Coll. Cardiol.*, **6**, 653–662

12. GOLDBERG, S. J., SAHN, D. J., ALLEN, H. D., VALDES-CRUZ, L. M., HOENECKE, H. and CARNAHAN, Y. (1982) Evaluation of pulmonary and systemic blood flow by two-dimensional Doppler echocardiography using fast Fourier transform spectral analysis. *Am. J. Cardiol.*, **50**, 1394–1400

13. SANDERS, S. P., YEAGER, S. and WILLIAMS, R. G. (1983) Measurement of systemic and pulmonary blood flow and QP/QS ratio using Doppler and two-dimensional echocardiography. *Am. J. Cardiol.*, **51**, 952–956

14. ORMINSTON, J. A., SHAH, P. M., TEI, C. and WONG, M. (1981) Size and motion of the mitral valve annulus in man. A two-dimensional echocardiographic method and findings in normal subjects. *Circulation*, **64**, 113–120

15. FISHER, D. C., SAHN, D. J., FRIEDMAN, J. J. *et al.* (1983) The mitral valve orifice method for non-invasive two-dimensional echo Doppler determinations of cardiac output. *Circulation*, **67**, 872–877

16. ZANG, Y., NITTER-HAUGE, S., IHLEN, H. and MYHRE, E. (1985) Doppler echocardiographic measurement of cardiac output using the mitral orifice method. *Br. Heart J.*, **53**, 130–136

17. GISVOLD, S. E. and BRUBAKK, A. D. (1982) Measurements of instantaneous blood flow velocity in the human aorta using pulsed ultrasound. *Cardiovasc. Res.*, **16**, 26–33

18. POWNER, D. J. and SNYDER, J. V. (1978) *In vitro* comparison of six commercially available thermodilution cardiac output systems. *Med. Ins.*, **12**, 122–127

19. MENDEL, D. (1974) *A Practice of Cardiac Catheterisation*, 2nd edn, pp. 327–337. Oxford: Blackwell Scientific Publications

20. MATRE, K., SEGADAL, L. and ENGEDAHL, H. (1985) Continuous measurement of aortic blood velocity, after cardiac surgery by means of an extractable Doppler ultrasound probe. *J. Biomed. Eng.*, **7**, 84–88

21. ELKEYAM, U., GARDIN, J. M., BERKLEY, R., HUGHES, C. A. and HENRY, W. L. (1983) The use of Doppler flow velocity measurement to assess the hemodynamic response to vasodilators in patients with heart failure. *Circulation*, **67**, 377–383

22. SCHUSTER, A. H. and NANDA, N. C. (1982) Doppler echocardiography and cardiac pacing. *PACE*, **5**, 607–612

Appendix

A commonly used method to calculate cardiac output is to multiply the time velocity integral (cm) (called stroke distance on p. 15) by the area (cm^2) across which flow occurs to provide an estimate of the stroke volume (cm^3). This is then multiplied by the heart rate (to give ml/minute) and divided by 1000 to give cardiac output (CO) in l/min. Thus

$$\text{Cardiac output (l/min)} = \frac{\text{area}(\text{cm}^2) \times \text{velocity integral}(\text{cm}) \times \text{heart rate}(\text{min}^{-1})}{1000}$$

As previously explained, the integral of the flow velocity curve is obtained by measuring the area under (or integrating) the curve either electronically or by planimetry. Dividing the integral by the flow time (ejection time when the measurements are made in the outflow part of the heart), the temporal mean velocity of the flow period is obtained. In other words, the integral (cm) equals the temporal mean velocity of the flow period (cm/s) multiplied by the flow time (s). Using either procedure, diastolic flow (or systolic at the level of the atrioventricular valves) should not be included in the calculations since it usually represents eddies, not net flow (*Figure 10.1*).

11

Colour Doppler flow mapping

Walter Duncan and Iain A. Simpson

Colour Doppler flow mapping has only recently been introduced[1–3] and represents a significant advance in the development of Doppler ultrasound. It should be remembered that clinical application of colour Doppler flow mapping remains in its infancy and a subject of continuing active research, and that it is currently in routine clinical practice in relatively few centres. This technique allows the spatial appreciation of flow velocities in relationship to structural detail imaged in real time and some colour Doppler images have been integrated throughout the chapters of this book to allow a fuller appreciation of the relative value of this technique in relation to spectral Doppler.

The purpose of this chapter is to provide a clinical perspective of the current areas of cardiology where colour Doppler is of value. It does not therefore attempt to provide a comprehensive list of the possible applications of colour Doppler flow mapping, rather to delineate areas where this technique is currently used clinically and to provide some insight into its future potential.

It is noteworthy that in the few major centres which have been involved in colour Doppler flow mapping since its inception and have developed most expertise in its application, the technique has been shown to be of considerable clinical value over a wide range of cardiological conditions. In particular, by the combination of spatial, structural and functional information in real time, its value in congenital heart disease is unparalleled and it is to be expected that over the next few years a rapid expansion of this technique will occur in many areas of cardiology.

Physical principles

When using colour Doppler flow mapping it is necessary to have some understanding of the underlying physical principles which allow the operator to appreciate the strengths and limitations of the technique. These are more fully described elsewhere[4].

The major problem in the development of colour Doppler flow mapping was to overcome the time constraints of acquiring such large amounts of Doppler information. In a single colour Doppler image there may be as many as 2000 separate sample points, and it is not possible to use spectral analysis of conventional pulsed Doppler at each since it requires around 10 ms to perform spectral Doppler at each sample position. Therefore, the technique of autocorrelation was developed for colour flow mapping to overcome this problem. Here, for each line of the colour sector, a number of successive ultrasound pulses are transmitted, known as the *pulse train* or *pulse packet size*. One pulse is used for tissue information and the Doppler information is acquired from the remaining pulses by comparison of the phase difference of successive pulses. The mean value is then matched, or autocorrelated, with a memory bank within the flow mapping equipment and a colour assigned for that particular velocity. Flow towards the transducer is generally assigned the colour red and flow away from the transducer blue, with increasing colour intensities indicating higher velocities. There is only a limited number of possibilities or colour intensities (generally 16 for red towards flow and 16 for blue away flow) which can be assigned for a particular velocity from 0 m/s to the Nyquist limit, which for most systems is around 0.5 m/s, depending on the pulse repetition frequency, and the system will choose the closest colour/mean velocity match.

Time constraints of colour Doppler flow mapping relate to the line density, the sector size, the depth or pulse repetition frequency, the frame rate and the number of pulses in the pulse train, and any modification of one of these will be a trade-off against another. For example, the quality of the Doppler information is related to the number of successive pulses analysed, but increasing the number of pulses will increase the time constraints and therefore result in a decrease in frame rate.

The flow mapping system will also use the successive pulses of the pulse train to calculate the statistical variation around the mean value, and if this 'variance' is above a certain level, indicative of turbulent flow, it will overlay green on the colour velocity assignment producing varying levels of turquoise and yellow. Disturbed or turbulent flow will then appear as a multicolour mosaic pattern. This variance display is extremely valuable in distinguishing between normal and abnormal flow patterns and, in particular, for identifying the origin and distribution of the turbulent high velocity jets associated with valvar stenosis or regurgitation.

It should be remembered that colour Doppler flow mapping systems are mean velocity estimators, and they are also pulsed Doppler systems and hence are subject to frequency aliasing. Frequency aliasing is a problem with conventional pulsed Doppler but appears to be advantageous for the application of colour Doppler flow mapping. Since, unlike conventional pulsed Doppler, colour Doppler allows spatial appreciation of flow velocities, the presence of colour aliasing can be useful in identifying high velocity laminar flow. For example, in mitral stenosis, the aliased (blue) central core of the high velocity laminar flow, with surrounding non-aliased red flow, is easily identified, indicating the presence of obstruction and separating this from the non-aliased, low velocity inflow pattern across a normal mitral valve. Also the spatial information provided by colour Doppler flow mapping allows appreciation of multiple aliasing patterns associated with rapidly accelerating flow not possible with conventional Doppler systems, and visualized spatially by successive blue/red changes in colour.

The major problem currently associated with colour Doppler imaging in comparison to imaging alone is the relatively slow frame rate, which is of particular importance in infants and children with rapid heart rates. In these patients, however, the frame rate can be optimized by coning down on the area of interest thereby reducing the colour sector size, by reducing the imaging depth resulting in increased pulse repetition frequency and, if necessary, by reducing the pulse packet size, although the latter will cause some degradation in the quality of Doppler information.

There is a tremendous amount of information contained within a single colour Doppler image and it may not be possible in some patients, even for an experienced operator, to appreciate all this information in real time, particularly when there are numerous or complex lesions and subsequent frame-by-frame video analysis will be required. When learning to interpret colour Doppler images the use of frame-by-frame analysis should be performed in all cases.

Orientation and normal flow patterns

Colour flow imaging is performed initially from the four standard cross-sectional echocardiographic planes: parasternal long and short axis, apical four chamber and suprasternal notch view. As with spectral Doppler, the position and angulation which provide the best echocardiographic images in standard views are not always those which are optimal for flow imaging and minor positional changes may be required depending on the requirements of the individual study.

The routine flow designation can vary between instruments but most frequently is assigned as:

Red = blood flow towards the transducer (a positive Doppler shift on spectral display)

Blue = blood flow away from the transducer (a negative Doppler shift on spectral display).

A colour bar at the margin of the display serves as a reminder of the colour/direction assigned. In some equipment a reversal switch is available to permit the opposite colour/direction assignment to be chosen if required.

The normal systolic and diastolic sequence in a long axis view produces red mitral diastolic inflow and blue systolic outflow along the left ventricular outflow tract in both parasternal (*see Plates 17a* and *b*) and apical (*see Plate 2*) views.

The parasternal short axis views are performed in an apex to base sweep similar to standard imaging. At the great artery level, normal tricuspid inflow (in red) shows a colour change as each volume of blood passes through the body of the right ventricle and the right ventricular outflow tract becomes blue as blood flows into the lungs (*see Plate 18*).

The apical four chamber (and five chamber) views show red diastolic inflow through both atrioventricular valves (*see Plate 19*), and demonstrate blue flow in the left ventricular outflow tract during systole.

Suprasternal notch imaging shows ascending aortic flow in red and blue flow in the descending aortic segment (*see Plate 20*).

Other scanning planes are chosen as necessary to provide optimal images of the flow patterns, particularly in congenital heart defects.

Clinical application of colour Doppler

The future clinical applications of colour Doppler flow mapping in both acquired and congenital heart disease will undoubtedly be extensive and the combination of real-time spatial flow velocity information with structural detail will allow an improved understanding of the pathophysiology and natural history of many cardiac lesions. Colour Doppler flow mapping remains in its infancy and the clinical applications of the technique remain unclear. However, initial findings in the use of colour Doppler have suggested that potentially the technique can be of value in the assessment of heart disease by applying it in several basic ways.

(1) Where an anatomical abnormality is of relatively small size or is poorly delineated by echocardiography because of the transmission characteristics of the tissue, colour Doppler may, by outlining boundaries of blood flow, enhance the two-dimensional echocardiographic image and provide anatomical information additional to that provided by conventional imaging on the site of specific lesions. Thus the demonstration of the site of flow, particularly when of high velocity with aliasing, will indicate the position of blood-filled spaces and demonstrate any anatomical defect through which it occurs even if it is too small to be apparent on echocardiography, e.g. a small septal defect, or the position and extent of regurgitant flow.

(2) Where a jet is picked up with continuous wave Doppler and could potentially come from more than one position along its length but its velocity is outside that which can be measured with pulsed or high pulse repetition frequency systems, colour imaging will show aliasing and thus indicate the position along the continuous wave beam at which this happens, e.g. distinguishing mitral regurgitation from aortic stenosis.

(3) Optimization of the alignment of the Doppler beam to flow should theoretically be possible since colour mapping shows the direction of a jet and not just the margins of the chambers and vessels. If after manipulation of transducer position and angulation it is not possible to align the beam and apparent jet within a 20° angle, the direction of each can be assessed and, depending on the preference of the operator, it can be accepted that the true velocity will be underestimated or correction for the angle of incidence can then be undertaken with greater confidence than with a simple imaging system.

(4) Better assessment of regurgitation may be provided since the flow will be apparent along all the lines in the colour flow image almost simultaneously giving an idea of the extent of the regurgitation in a complete plane and thus a two-dimensional demonstration of flow velocities.

It must always be borne in mind that colour Doppler, like two-dimensional echocardiography, only gives a single plane view and will miss higher velocities in another plane if care is not exercised in its use. Indeed, it may sometimes be easier to pick up the high velocity jet with continuous wave Doppler alone and, while keeping the transducer and beam on this, switch on imaging and colour to show its anatomical site. This technique is however the complete opposite to that generally advocated for the use of colour Doppler as a screening test, and each operator will have to decide with experience which is most appropriate for the individual needs of the patient and the cardiology department. It is perhaps best to consider conventional and colour Doppler as complementary (as are M-mode and two-dimensional echocardiography) and use each as seems most appropriate to obtain the optimal study.

Colour Doppler in adult cardiology

In adult cardiology practice Doppler has its main application in:

the assessment of the severity of stenosis
the estimation of the severity of regurgitation
the quantitation of cardiac output.

It is therefore appropriate to consider the use of colour Doppler in each of these applications. When studying large subjects, particularly with dilated hearts, it is worthwhile remembering that colour Doppler can suffer to some extent from a reduction in sensitivity with increasing depth and in some situations the transducer will have to be moved to bring the area of interest closer to it.

In Chapters 4 and 5 the assessment of stenosis has briefly alluded to the use of colour Doppler. Colour can clearly show the site of the lesion and origin of the high velocity jet. However, in aortic stenosis the colour signal tends to show a mosaic of colours in the entire area just distal to the obstruction and a clear jet as seen on angiocardiography is not apparent. Thus with aortic stenosis it is still advisiable to examine all positions with stand alone continuous wave Doppler to obtain the optimal signal which often requires the use of sites which are not suitable for imaging and colour Doppler. The use of colour Doppler and angle correction is fraught with problems and should not be used unless there is no alternative because of poor imaging characteristics of the subject.

However, in some lesions, particularly with prosthetic valves, the direction of flow may be such that it is very difficult to obtain good alignment and colour Doppler will then allow angle correction (*see Plates 3* and *16*) which may be of value in obtaining the most accurate measurement of gradient. Colour Doppler can be of assistance in aligning the beam along the direction of the regurgitant jet through the atrioventricular and semilunar valves. This can be of considerable value in attempting to assess pulmonary (or right ventricular) pressure.

Colour Doppler is superior to mapping with pulsed Doppler in the assessment of regurgitant lesions (*see Plates 1, 4, 5, 6, 7, 8, 9* and *10*) and allows clearer demonstration of the extent of the regurgitation flow velocities. However, initial studies would indicate that the regurgitant jet area on colour flow mapping provides only a semiquantitative assessment of the severity of mitral regurgitation[5, 6]. The velocity distribution of regurgitant jets may well be dependent on a number of factors including haemodynamic variables[7] and much work is still required to determine the exact significance of colour Doppler flow mapping in valvar regurgitation. Again, it must be remembered that only a single plane is visualized, that the apparent extent can be affected by gain settings and, where there is a relatively large distance from the transducer to flow area, artefacts in flow velocities in the near field can occur. Although the extent of the regurgitant flow is useful information, in itself, it is not the major determinant of the clinical significance of the effect of the lesion and the need for surgery. Exact localization of the origin of the regurgitant jet will assist in the study of prosthetic valves to determine whether flow is through the valve itself or in the paravalve area, but the penetration problems of ultrasound through mechanical prostheses encountered with conventional Doppler techniques also pertain to colour Doppler flow mapping[8].

Colour Doppler techniques are as yet not sufficiently sensitive to demonstrate the flow profile across the vessel and allow prediction of the most appropriate position from which to record the flow signal to provide the spatial mean velocity. However, the use of different colour Doppler algorithms including the power mode, which enhances the sensitivity of colour Doppler for low velocity flow, may provide a clearer demonstration of the area through which flow occurs; measurement of this area is the most difficult (and potentially inaccurate) factor to obtain for the measurement of cardiac output.

Colour Doppler in congenital heart disease

Colour flow imaging in children can produce a dramatically clear and accurate demonstration of intra- and extracardiac flow. The relatively short beam penetration depth required in concert with less calcified ribs and large heart produces clear blood flow imaging with little artefactual interference at the highest available pulse repetition frequency.

Ideally, a 5.0 MHz probe should be used for most imaging of cardiac structure and flow in patients in the first few years of life and a 3.5 MHz probe for older children. However, the higher frequency transducer has a relatively low aliasing velocity and in some instances the use of a lower frequency probe with its higher aliasing velocity can provide better quality Doppler information.

In some centres colour flow imaging is used as a screening tool for all new patients who are undergoing an initial echocardiographic examination. For patients with a documented flow abnormality, range-gated pulsed Doppler and/or continuous wave Doppler is then utilized further to delineate the flow disturbance and, if necessary, measure the maximum velocity.

The same basic principles in the use of colour Doppler apply equally well to congenital as to acquired heart disease. Doppler is likely to have its main application in:

demonstration of the presence and site of defects
assessment of the severity of stenosis
measurement of pulmonary artery pressure.

The technique may be of particular value in the demonstration of the sites of abnormal flow, thus confirming the presence of small defects which are not apparent on echocardiography. This is most easily seen with the ventricular septal defect (VSD). A defect of haemodynamic significance is virtually always demonstrable with echocardiography and the spectral signal can be recognized without colour Doppler even with a non-imaging system. Colour Doppler may allow the VSD site to be recognized more quickly and simply demonstrates the flow dynamics across it as shown in *Plates 11a* and *b* in a parasternal view of an infant with a moderately large subaortic (perimembranous) VSD who had already undergone pulmonary artery banding as palliative surgery. The bidirectional nature of the shunt flow in this particular case was demonstrated as flow from the left ventricular outflow tract into the right ventricle (red) and later from right ventricle to aorta (blue).

It seems that, in VSD, colour Doppler may be of particular value in confirming the presence and site of small defects. This is apparent in studies of a child with a small muscular VSD shown in *Plate 12*. Continuous wave Doppler showed only a short atypical early systolic signal while colour Doppler clearly demonstrated the defect and flow through it. This is also shown in *Plate 13*, from a young man who developed a VSD murmur following a left parasternal stab wound, but in whom the VSD was not found with imaging echocardiography alone.

In patients with a ductus arteriosus, particularly the preterm infant with lung disease requiring ventilation, the region of the ductus arteriosus may be quite difficult to visualize and the accurate diagnosis of ductal patency by direct visualization is dubious. Doppler can usually demonstrate the typical spectral signal. However, this signal can be atypical and it can be particularly difficult to obtain typical good quality spectral signals in ventilated babies. Colour Doppler can then make recognition of ductal flow much simpler, as shown in a 1200 g infant in *Plate 14*; normal antegrade pulmonary artery flow is shown in blue with the reversed or retrograde ductal flow in red. This of course only confirms the presence of the ductus arteriosus and further studies are required to ascertain whether Doppler adds anything to the simple measurement of the ratio of the left atrium to aorta in determining the need for surgical closure in the preterm infant. As discussed in Chapter 8 the colour flow demonstration of flow through the ductus arteriosus into the main pulmonary artery is of particular value in those with an atypical murmur in whom the spectral signal is also atypical and without Doppler there may be need for diagnostic catheterization.

Doppler is not usually required to confirm the presence of a significant atrial septal defect (ASD), but a Doppler study, colour or spectral, showing no flow across the atrial septum virtually excludes a left to right shunt at atrial level. Even a small shunt through a patent foramen ovale or a tiny ASD can be shown by colour Doppler (*Plate 15*).

Continuous wave Doppler can obtain good signals to measure the gradient in younger patients with pulmonary or aortic valve stenosis and colour flow has little to add. However, where the obstruction occurs at another position, colour can demonstrate its site.

Assessment of pulmonary pressure requires measurement of the velocity of tricuspid or pulmonary regurgitation or pressure drop across the ventricular septum. Colour demonstration of the flow direction will help in aligning the spectral beam (*Plates 6* and *9*), but it is not yet certain whether careful examination with colour or continuous wave stand alone Doppler is more accurate in finding these very small, often high velocity, jets.

Intraoperative colour Doppler

Use of intraoperative echocardiography has followed the same transitional pathway as precordial echocardiography. The inital use of M-mode studies to look at cardiac wall motion was followed by cross-sectional ultrasound used in many reports of surgery for many types of cardiac anomalies[10]. More recently, colour flow imaging has been applied intraoperatively following valve repairs and replacement, congenital cardiac repairs and aortic ancurysm resections[11].

For intraoperative use the probe can be gas sterilized or a sterile plastic bag can be used to cover the probe. Its use is illustrated in *Plates 21a* and *b* from a 12-year-old boy who had mitral regurgitation 2 years after mitral valve replacement. Standard colour flow Doppler imaging and cardiac catheterization suggested a significant regurgitant volume and repeat surgery was undertaken. After surgical repair of two atrioventricular fistulous tracts in the periannular tissue adjacent to the prosthetic sewing ring, the patient was weaned from cardiopulmonary bypass. Colour flow imaging performed from a modified four-chamber view revealed a persistent regurgitant jet in the periannular region (*see Plate 21a*). The surgical site was re-explored and a third fistulous communication was discovered and probed. This was oversewn and bypass again discontinued. Colour flow imaging showed no persistence of the periannular regurgitation (*see Plate 21b*). The patient has subsequently done well.

Conclusions

The development of colour Doppler flow mapping is a significant and exciting advance in non-invasive imaging. The dynamic appreciation of spatial flow velocity information combined with high resolution tissue imaging confers considerable potential for this technique in the study of a variety of cardiological conditions. Its valuable clinical role is rapidly becoming established in the assessment of congenital heart lesions where the combination of structural and functional information is particularly important, and a considerable number of applications in adult cardiology are also becoming apparent.

Its role should be regarded as complementary to echocardiography and conventional Doppler ultrasound and, in particular, the use of colour flow directed continuous wave Doppler is likely to enhance the ease of application of this technique and lessen the potential error in gradient estimation encountered with conventional image directed or stand alone continuous wave Doppler. Much research is required in the area of colour Doppler flow mapping. Although the ability to provide qualitative information in many cardiological lesions is clear, further investigation is needed to establish its role in quantitative asessment. For example, it is easy to appreciate the presence of a regurgitant jet by colour Doppler, but the way in which the spatial velocity information it provides relates to the quantitative assessment of regurgitation and to the effect of haemodynamic changes on colour Doppler regurgitant jets, remains to be established. As with spectral Doppler, colour assignment on colour Doppler flow mapping is angle dependent, and it may be that future advances will allow the display of angle independent velocities, and the manner of display of the vast amount of flow velocity information contained in a single colour Doppler image may be radically altered.

It has been suggested that colour Doppler flow mapping is more easily performed than conventional spectral Doppler and will aid general acceptance of the technique. While it is true that the integration of structural information makes orientation easier, a considerable and particular expertise is required not only in acquiring but also interpreting colour Doppler information, and it should not be expected that a person experienced in two-dimensional imaging will be able to develop an expertise in colour Doppler flow mapping without a significant learning curve.

With continuing advances in colour Doppler technology, it is likely that colour Doppler flow mapping will play an increasingly important role in the assessment of both adult and congenital heart disease in clinical cardiological practice.

References

1. OMOTO, R., YOKOTE, Y., TAKAMOTO, S. *et al.* (1984) The development of real-time two-dimensional Doppler echocardiography and its clinical significance in acquired valvular disease. *Jpn. Heart J.*, **25**, 325–340

2. MIYATAKE, K., OKAMOTO, M., KINOSHITA, N. *et al.* (1984) Clinical applications of a new type of real-time two-dimensional Doppler flow imaging system. *Am. J. Cardiol.*, **54**, 857–868

3. SAHN, D. J. (1985) Real-time two-dimensional Doppler echocardiography flow mapping. *Circulation*, **71**, 849–853

4. OMOTO, R. and KASAI, C. (1986) Basic principles of Doppler color flow imaging. Echocardiography: a review of cardiovascular ultrasound. **3**, 463–473

5. MIYATAKE, K., IZUMI, S., OKAMOTO, M. *et al.* (1986) Semiquantitative grading of severity of mitral regurgitation by real-time two-dimensional Doppler flow imaging technique. *J. Am. Coll. Cardiol.,* **7,** 82–86

6. HELMCKE, F., NANDA, N. C., HSIUNG, M. C. *et al.* (1987) Color Doppler assessment of mitral regurgitation with orthogonal planes. *Circulation,* **75,** 175–183

7. SWITZER, D. F., YOGANATHAN, A. P., NANDA, N. C., WOO, Y. and RIDWAY, A. J. (1987) Calibration of colour Doppler flow mapping during extreme hemodynamic conditions *in vitro:* a foundation for a reliable quantitative grading system for aortic incompetence. *Circulation,* **75,** 837–846

8. SPRECHER, D. L., ADAMICK, R., ADAMS, D. and KISSLO, J. (1987) *In vitro* color flow, pulsed and continuous wave Doppler ultrasound masking of flow by prosthetic valves. *J. Am. Coll. Cardiol.,* **9,** 1306–1310

9. SWENSSON, R. E., VALDES-CRUZ, L. M., SAHN, D. J. *et al.* (1986) Real-time Doppler color flow mapping for detection of patent ductus arteriosus. *J. Am. Coll. Cardiol.,* **8,** 1105–1112

10. GOLDMAN, M. E. and MINDICH, B. P. (1986) Intraoperative two-dimensional Doppler echocardiography: new application of an old technique. *J. Am. Coll. Cardiol.,* **7,** 374–382

11. TAKAMOTO, S., KYO, S., ADACHI, H., MATSURMA, M., HOKOTE, Y. and OMOTO, R. (1985) Intraoperative colour flow mapping by real-time two-dimensional Doppler echocardiography for evaluation of valvular and congenital heart disease and vascular disease. *J. Thorac. Cardiovasc. Surg,* **79,** 802–812

Index

345 137
2/2/89